# RN Community Health Nu

## REVIEW MODULE EDITION 7.0

## Contributors

Norma Jean E. Henry, MSN/Ed, RN

Mendy McMichael, DNP, MSN

Janean Johnson, MSN, RN, CNE

Agnes DiStasi, DNP, RN, CNE

Carrie B. Elkins, DHSc, MSN

Honey C. Holman, MSN, RN

## Consultants

Deb Johnson-Schuh, RN, MSN, CNE

Jenni L. Hoffman, DNP, FNP-C, CLNC

*Director of content review: Kristen Lawler*

*Director of development: Derek Prater*

*Project management: Janet Hines, Nicole Burke*

*Coordination of content review: Norma Jean E. Henry, Mendy McMichael*

*Copy editing: Kelly Von Lunen, Derek Prater*

*Layout: Spring Lenox, Randi Hardy*

*Illustrations: Randi Hardy*

*Online media: Morgan Smith, Ron Hanson, Nicole Lobdell, Brant Stacy*

*Cover design: Jason Buck*

*Interior book design: Spring Lenox*

## IMPORTANT NOTICE TO THE READER

# User's Guide

Welcome to the Assessment Technologies Institute® RN Community Health Nursing Review Module Edition 7.0. The mission of ATI's Content Mastery Series® Review Modules is to provide user-friendly compendiums of nursing knowledge that will:
- Help you locate important information quickly.
- Assist in your learning efforts.
- Provide exercises for applying your nursing knowledge.
- Facilitate your entry into the nursing profession as a newly licensed nurse.

This newest edition of the Review Modules has been redesigned to optimize your learning experience. We've fit more content into less space and have done so in a way that will make it even easier for you to find and understand the information you need.

## ORGANIZATION

Chapters in this Review Module use a nursing concepts organizing framework, beginning with an overview describing the central concept and its relevance to nursing. Subordinate themes are covered in outline form to demonstrate relationships and present the information in a clear, succinct manner. Some chapters have sections that group related concepts and contain their own overviews. These sections are included in the table of contents.

## ACTIVE LEARNING SCENARIOS AND APPLICATION EXERCISES

Each chapter includes opportunities for you to test your knowledge and to practice applying that knowledge. Active Learning Scenario exercises pose a nursing scenario and then direct you to use an ATI Active Learning Template (included at the back of this book) to record the important knowledge a nurse should apply to the scenario. An example is then provided to which you can compare your completed Active Learning Template. The Application Exercises include NCLEX-style questions, such as multiple-choice and multiple-select items, providing you with opportunities to practice answering the kinds of questions you might expect to see on ATI assessments or the NCLEX. After the Application Exercises, an answer key is provided, along with rationales.

## NCLEX® CONNECTIONS

To prepare for the NCLEX-RN, it is important to understand how the content in this Review Module is connected to the NCLEX-RN test plan. You can find information on the detailed test plan at the National Council of State Boards of Nursing's website, www.ncsbn.org. When reviewing content in this Review Module, regularly ask yourself, "How does this content fit into the test plan, and what types of questions related to this content should I expect?"

To help you in this process, we've included NCLEX Connections at the beginning of each unit and with each question in the Application Exercises Answer Keys. The NCLEX Connections at the beginning of each unit point out areas of the detailed test plan that relate to the content within that unit. The NCLEX Connections attached to the Application Exercises Answer Keys demonstrate how each exercise fits within the detailed content outline. These NCLEX Connections will help you understand how the detailed content outline is organized, starting with major client needs categories and subcategories and followed by related content areas and tasks. The major client needs categories are:
- Safe and Effective Care Environment
  - Management of Care
  - Safety and Infection Control
- Health Promotion and Maintenance
- Psychosocial Integrity
- Physiological Integrity
  - Basic Care and Comfort
  - Pharmacological and Parenteral Therapies
  - Reduction of Risk Potential
  - Physiological Adaptation

An NCLEX Connection might, for example, alert you that content within a unit is related to:
- Safety and Infection Control
  - Home Safety
    - Assess need for client home modifications.

## QSEN COMPETENCIES

As you use the Review Modules, you will note the integration of the Quality and Safety Education for Nurses (QSEN) competencies throughout the chapters. These competencies are integral components of the curriculum of many nursing programs in the United States and prepare you to provide safe, high-quality care as a newly licensed nurse. Icons appear to draw your attention to the six QSEN competencies.

**Safety:** The minimization of risk factors that could cause injury or harm while promoting quality care and maintaining a secure environment for clients, self, and others.

**Patient-Centered Care:** The provision of caring and compassionate, culturally sensitive care that addresses clients' physiological, psychological, sociological, spiritual, and cultural needs, preferences, and values.

**Evidence-Based Practice:** The use of current knowledge from research and other credible sources, on which to base clinical judgment and client care.

**Informatics:** The use of information technology as a communication and information-gathering tool that supports clinical decision-making and scientifically based nursing practice.

**Quality Improvement:** Care related and organizational processes that involve the development and implementation of a plan to improve health care services and better meet clients' needs.

**Teamwork and Collaboration:** The delivery of client care in partnership with multidisciplinary members of the health care team to achieve continuity of care and positive client outcomes.

## ICONS

Icons are used throughout the Review Module to draw your attention to particular areas. Keep an eye out for these icons.

**(N)** This icon is used for NCLEX Connections.

**(G)** This icon indicates gerontological considerations, or knowledge specific to the care of older adult clients.

**Qs** This icon is used for content related to safety and is a QSEN competency. When you see this icon, take note of safety concerns or steps that nurses can take to ensure client safety and a safe environment.

**Qpcc** This icon is a QSEN competency that indicates the importance of a holistic approach to providing care.

**Qebp** This icon, a QSEN competency, points out the integration of research into clinical practice.

**Qi** This icon is a QSEN competency and highlights the use of information technology to support nursing practice.

**Qqi** This icon is used to focus on the QSEN competency of integrating planning processes to meet clients' needs.

**Qtc** This icon highlights the QSEN competency of care delivery using an interprofessional approach.

**M◇** This icon appears at the top-right of pages and indicates availability of an online media supplement, such as a graphic, animation, or video. If you have an electronic copy of the Review Module, this icon will appear alongside clickable links to media supplements. If you have a hard copy version of the Review Module, visit www.atitesting.com for details on how to access these features.

## FEEDBACK

ATI welcomes feedback regarding this Review Module. Please provide comments to comments@atitesting.com.

# Table of Contents

When reviewing the following chapter, keep in mind the relevant topics and tasks of the NCLEX outline, in particular:

## Client Needs: Management of Care

**ADVOCACY:** Utilize advocacy resources appropriately.

**ETHICAL PRACTICE:** Practice in a manner consistent with the code of ethics for registered nurses.

## Client Needs: Health Promotion and Maintenance

**HEALTH PROMOTION/DISEASE PREVENTION:** Educate the client on actions to promote/maintain health and prevent disease.

**HEALTH SCREENING:** Perform targeted screening assessments (e.g., vision, nutrition).

upstream thinking is
concerned w/ prevention.
and promoting health.

HEALTH BOARDS: monitor disease, promote health,
and collect statistics about the community.

UPSTREAM THINKING: prevention of disease and
health promotion.

Overview of Community Health Nursing

Community health nursing is a population-focused approach to planning, delivering, and evaluating nursing care. Community health nursing is a broad field that allows nurses to practice in a wide variety of settings. Community health nurses promote the health and welfare of clients across the lifespan and from diverse populations.

Nurses working in the community should have an understanding of the foundations of community health nursing, the principles guiding community health nursing, epidemiology, and health promotion and disease prevention.

# Foundations of community health nursing

- Concepts related to public health are evident throughout history as provisions were made to care for the poor or displaced. Advances in knowledge about health led to appropriate education of providers and regulation of water and other environmental factors.
- The Public Health Service was developed in 1798, and nursing care in homes was implemented in the early 1800s. Later in the century, efforts began to establish local health boards to monitor disease, promote health, and collect statistics about the community.
- Various theories and specific definitions of care guide nursing practice in the community.

*Systems thinking: cause/effect relationships.*

## COMMUNITY HEALTH NURSING THEORIES

- **Systems thinking** studies how an individual, or unit, interacts with other organizations or systems. Systems thinking is useful in examining cause and effect relationships.
- **Upstream thinking** is used to focus on interventions that promote health or prevent illness, as opposed to medical treatment models that focus on care after an individual becomes ill.
- Nursing theory provides the basis for care of the community and family. Theorists have developed sound principles to guide nurses in providing high-quality care. Examples of nursing theories appropriate for community health include the following.

*Nightingale: relationship b/w environment + health. health is a continuum.*

### Nightingale's Environmental Theory

- Highlights the relationship between an individual's environment and health.
- Depicts health as a continuum.
- Emphasizes preventive care.

### Health Belief Model *individual.*

- Purpose is to predict or explain health behaviors.
- Assumes that preventive health behaviors are taken primarily for the purpose of avoiding disease.
- Emphasizes change at the individual level.
- Describes the likelihood of taking an action to avoid disease based on the following.
  - Perceived susceptibility, seriousness, and threat of a disease
  - Modifying factors (e.g., demographics, knowledge level)
  - Cues to action (e.g., media campaigns, disease effect on family/friends, recommendations from health care professionals)
  - Perceived benefits minus perceived barriers to taking action

### Milio's framework for prevention *community.*

- Complements the health belief model.
- Emphasizes change at the community level.
- Identifies relationship between health deficits and availability of health-promoting resources.
- Theorizes that behavior changes within a large number of people can ultimately lead to social change.

### Pender's Health Promotion Model

- Similar to Health Belief Model.
- Does not consider health risk as a factor that provokes change.
- Examines factors that affect individual actions to promote and protect health.
  - Personal factors (biological, psychological, sociocultural), behaviors, abilities, self-efficacy
  - Feelings, benefits, barriers, and characteristics associated with the action
  - Attitudes of others, and competing demands and preferences

## ESSENTIALS OF COMMUNITY NURSING

- **Determinants of health** are factors that influence the client's health. These can include nutrition, stress, education, the environment, finances, and social status/stigma (prejudice).
- **Health indicators** (mortality rates, disease prevalence, levels of physical activity, obesity, tobacco or other substance use) describe the health status of a community and serve as targets for the improvement of a community's health.
- **Nurses** determine a community's health by examining the degree to which the community's collective health needs are identified and met.

- **Community** is a group of people and institutions that share geographic, civic, and/or social parameters. Communities vary in their characteristics and health needs.
- Community health nursing involves a synthesis of nursing and public health theory.
- The goals of community health nursing are to promote, preserve, and maintain the health of populations by the delivery of health services to individuals, families, and groups in order to influence "community health."
- Community health nurses are nurses who practice in the community. They usually have a facility from which they work (community health clinic, county health department), but their practice is not limited to institutional settings. Care is often delivered in a setting that is part of the client's environment (home, school, workplace).
- The community or a population (an aggregate who shares one or more personal characteristics) within the community is the "client" in community health nursing. Q̇PCC
- Community health nurses can develop long-term relationships with clients while working directly with families and groups over a long period of time.

## Public health nursing

- Public health nursing is population-focused, and involves a combination of nursing knowledge along with social and public health sciences. The goal of public health nursing is promoting health and preventing disease.
- Public health provides 10 essential services, one of which is to conduct research to gain new knowledge and solutions to public health problems. The remainder fall under the three core functions of public health, according to www.cdc.gov.

ASSESSMENT: Using systematic methods to monitor the health of a population
- Monitor health status to identify community health problems.
- Diagnose and investigate health problems and health hazards in the community.

PUBLIC HEALTH NURSING 3 CORE FUNCTIONS:
Assessment.¹  Policy development.²  assurance.³

POLICY DEVELOPMENT: Developing laws and practices to promote the health of a population based on scientific evidence
- Inform, educate, and empower people about health issues.
- Mobilize community partnerships to identify and solve health problems.
- Develop policies and plans that support individual and community health efforts.

ASSURANCE: Making sure adequate health care personnel and services are accessible, especially to those who might not normally have them Q̇QI
- Enforce laws and regulations that protect health and ensure safety.
- Link people to needed personal health services and ensure the provision of health care when otherwise unavailable.
- Ensure a competent public health and personal health care workforce.
- Evaluate effectiveness, accessibility, and quality of personal and population-based health services.

## Population-focused nursing

- Population-focused nursing includes assessing to determine needs, intervening to protect and promote health, and preventing disease within a specific population (individuals at risk for hypertension, individuals without health insurance, individuals with a specific knowledge deficit).
- The Public Health Intervention Wheel is a widely used model for public health interventions and is available through the Minnesota Department of Health at www.health.state.mn.us.
- Community partnership occurs when community members, agencies, and businesses actively participate in the processes of health promotion and disease prevention. The development of community partnerships is critical to the accomplishment of health promotion and disease prevention strategies.

KEY PRINCIPLES OF PUBLIC HEALTH NURSING
- Emphasize primary prevention.
- Work to achieve the greatest good for the largest number of individuals.
- Recognize that the client is a partner in health.
- Use resources wisely to promote the best outcomes.

### 1.1 Community health nursing

| | | Community-oriented nursing | Community-based nursing |
|---|---|---|---|
| FOCUS OF CARE | | Aggregates, communities, populations (public health) Can include at-risk or unserved individuals and families | Individuals and families |
| PRIMARY GOAL | | Health promotion and disease prevention | Management of acute or chronic conditions |
| NURSING ACTIVITIES | | Usually indirect (program management) Can include direct care of at-risk individuals and populations | Direct (one-on-one) Illness care: Management of acute and chronic conditions in settings where individuals, families, and groups live, work, and "attend" (schools, camps, prisons) |

# Principles guiding community health nursing*

Factors to consider when providing community health nursing practice include the following.
- Ethics
- Advocacy
- Evidence-based practice
- Quality
- Professional collaboration and communication

## ETHICS

- The Public Health Code of Ethics identifies the ethical practice of public health. Ethical considerations include preventing harm, doing no harm, promoting good, respecting both individual and community rights, respecting autonomy and diversity, and providing confidentiality, competency, trustworthiness, and advocacy.
- Community health nurses are concerned with protecting, promoting, preserving, and maintaining health, as well as preventing disease. These concerns reflect the ethical principle of promoting good and preventing harm. Balancing individual rights vs. rights of community groups is a challenge.
- Community health nurses address the challenges of autonomy and providing ethical care. Client rights include the right to information disclosure, privacy, informed consent, information confidentiality, and participation in treatment decisions.
- As nurses participate in research in the community setting, it is important to use ethical decision-making to promote client rights.
- Public health nurses can apply ethical principles through core functions as they collect and manage information (assessment), develop policies that are in the best interest of the people in an area (policy development), and create interventions that promote healthcare equality across population groups (assurance).

*Balancing individual rights and community rights is difficult*

## ADVOCACY

Client advocate is one role of the community health nurse. The nurse plays the role of informer, supporter, and mediator for the client. The following are basic to client advocacy.
- Clients are autonomous beings who have the right to make decisions affecting their own health and welfare.
- Clients have the right to expect a nurse–client relationship that is based on trust, collaboration, and shared respect; related to health; and considerate of their thoughts and feelings.
- Clients are responsible for their own health.
- It is the nurse's responsibility to advocate for resources or services that meet the client's health care needs.
- Advocating for clients requires assertiveness, placing priority on the client's values, and willingness to progress through the chain of command for resolution.
- Nurses act as advocates for communities and populations through efforts to change health care systems and improve quality of life. An example of public health advocacy includes nurses working to promote access to clinics for individuals who live in rural communities.

### 1.2 Application of ethical principles to community health nursing

*Respect for autonomy*
Individuals select those actions that fulfill their goals.

SITUATIONS: Respecting a client's right to self-determination (making a decision not to pursue chemotherapy)

*Nonmaleficence*
No harm is done when applying standards of care.

SITUATIONS: Developing plans of care that include a system for monitoring and evaluating outcomes

*Beneficence*
Maximize possible benefits and minimize possible harms.

SITUATIONS: Assessing costs, risks and benefits when planning interventions

*Distributive justice*
Fair distribution of the benefits and burden in society is based on the needs and contributions of its members.

SITUATIONS: Determining eligibility for health care services based on income and fiscal resources

## EVIDENCE-BASED PRACTICE

Evidence-based practice involves using best practices, expert opinion, and client preferences to change the delivery of client care. The goal is to improve client outcomes.

### Data *consistency - results can be recreated.*

- The nurse should appraise data collected from research to measure whether bias was minimal (**quality**), the number of studies, participants, or strength of effect (**quantity**) and whether the results are repeatable (**consistency**). The nurse then analyzes the data for application to practice.
- Data is also classified to determine the strength of the information. The nurse should seek the highest level of evidence available and choose information that is validated by systematic peer-review.

### In the community

- Evidence-based practice improves public health as nurses develop policies to improve the health of specific groups. The public health nurse can use evidence to provide new solutions for groups of people (assessment), provide information to communities (policy development) and evaluate the effectiveness of the health care environment for groups (assurance).
- An example of evidence-based practice in community health includes the use of high levels of evidence to support media campaigns regarding immunization guidelines.

- The Task Force on Community Preventive Services produces a guide that reviews health promotion and disease prevention guidelines compared to the available evidence. The task force then determines whether there is sufficient or strong evidence to implement an intervention and lists which ones have insufficient evidence to show that they are effective.
- The nurse must consider several factors when applying evidence to practice: cost, benefit to the client, client satisfaction, safety, and client specific factors, such as culture and demographics. An intervention that is appropriate on the client or family level might not work when the nurse is caring for communities or populations of people.
- Nurses in the community setting can contribute to the body of evidence by implementing research studies in the practice setting and in collaboration with educational institutions, health care facilities, and through community-based participatory research (CBPR).
  - CBPR includes partners, professionals, and community residents in identifying health issues and intervening.
  - The CBPR approach fosters support from community members, develops leadership within the community, and promotes a positive collaborative relationship with health professionals.

# QUALITY

- Quality assurance, quality improvement, and quality management are part of improvement of health care. Detailed information about quality improvement is available in the **NURSING LEADERSHIP AND MANAGEMENT REVIEW MODULE**.
- Quality care is promoted through licensure and credentialing of health care providers, adherence to facility policies, professional development, and compliance with legal guidelines. Specialty certification is available for many community health roles.
- Quality report cards for managed care and public health organizations provide data about the effectiveness of care. Community health report cards can include health profiles, needs assessments, information about quality of life and health status.
- Nurses can use information from quality report cards in developing or revising strategies for care of communities. An example of increasing quality in community health is educating clients who have diabetes mellitus on how frequently their provider should perform glycosylated hemoglobin testing.

## Total quality management (TQM)

TQM is an approach that seeks to improve quality and performance which meets or exceeds expectations.

## Continuous quality improvement (CQI)

- CQI is an approach to quality management that emphasizes the organization and its processes and systems and uses objective data to analyze and improve processes.
- Public health nurses follow the continuous quality improvement process in carrying out roles of assessment, assurance, and policy development on an ongoing basis. Nurses can evaluate quality by examining the following aspects of care.
  - **Effectiveness:** providing services to those who will benefit
  - **Timeliness:** reducing waits and harmful delays in providing and receiving care
  - **Client-centered:** ensuring client values guide decision-making
  - **Equity:** providing equal care without discriminating against gender, race, sexual orientation, socioeconomic status
  - **Safety:** avoiding injuries to clients from the care intended to help them
  - **Efficiency:** avoiding waste in supplies, ideas, or energy

# PROFESSIONAL COLLABORATION AND COMMUNICATION

- Nurses in various community settings use communication skills in caring for individuals, collaborating in teams and groups, interacting with other professionals, and informing the public and stakeholders.
- The nurse facilitates communication with the client through transfers from one level of care to another, across the continuum of care.
- Nurse leaders use professional communication in roles such as mentoring, coaching employees, managing conflict, and supervising programs.
- Community health nurses should take care to use clear language with a respectful tone when using written, electronic, or print correspondence.
- The nurse should incorporate knowledge about variations in verbal and nonverbal communication, literacy needs, and client preferences when interacting with clients and groups.
- As with all aspects of health care, the nurse in the community setting is bound by laws regulating privacy and confidentiality in all forms of communication.

### BENEFITS OF PROFESSIONAL COMMUNICATION
- Increased client adherence to prescribed treatment plan
- Reduced admissions to acute care
- Reduced cost of care
- Shared decision-making with client and family
- Reduced medication errors

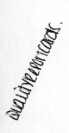

# COMMUNITY HEALTH EDUCATION

Community health nurses regularly provide health education in order to promote, maintain, and restore the health of populations. This is accomplished through a variety of means, such as community education programs.

In designing community education programs, nurses must take into account the barriers that make learning difficult. Some of these obstacles include age, cultural barriers, poor reading and comprehension skills, language barriers, barriers to access, and lack of motivation. Effective community health education requires planning. Qᴘᴄᴄ

## LEARNING THEORIES

**Behavioral theory:** Use of reinforcement methods to change learners' behaviors

**Cognitive theory:** Use of sensory input and repetition to change learners' patterns of thought, thereby changing behaviors

**Critical theory:** Use of ongoing discussion and inquiry to increase learners' depth of knowledge, thereby changing thinking and behaviors

**Developmental theory:** Use of techniques specific to learners' developmental stages to determine readiness to learn, and to impart knowledge

**Humanistic theory:** Assists learners to grow by emphasizing emotions and relationships and believing that free choice will prompt actions that are in their own best interest

**Social learning theory:** Links information to beliefs and values to change or shift the learners' expectations

## LEARNING STYLES

Community health nurses enhance the provision of education by addressing learning styles and domains of learning.

**Visual learners:** Learn through seeing and methods such as note taking, video viewing, and presentations. These learners "think in pictures."

**Auditory learners:** Learn through listening and methods such as verbal lectures, discussion, and reading aloud. These learners "interpret meaning while listening."

**Tactile-kinesthetic learners:** Learn through doing and methods such as trial and error, hands-on approaches, and return demonstration. These learners gain "meaning through exploration." *gain meaning through exploration.*

## DOMAINS OF LEARNING

**Cognitive domain:** Involves knowledge and the development of intellectual skills; for example a client discusses how sodium intake will affect blood pressure.

**Affective domain:** Involves a change in attitude and development of values; for example a client expresses acceptance of having a colostomy and maintains self-esteem.

**Psychomotor domain:** Involves the performance of a skill; for example, the community nurse teaches a client how to self-administer insulin.

# DEVELOPMENT OF A COMMUNITY HEALTH EDUCATION PLAN

- First, identify population-specific learning needs. Qᴏı
- Consider population-specific concerns and effects of health needs on the population to determine the priority learning need.
- Select aspects of learning theories (behavioral, cognitive, critical, developmental, humanistic, social learning) to use in the educational program based on the identified learning need.
- Identify barriers to learning, and learning styles (visual, auditory, tactile-kinesthetic).
- Design the educational program.
  - Set short- and long-term learning objectives that are measurable and achievable.
  - Select an appropriate educational method based on learning objectives and assessment of participants' learning styles.
  - Ensure written educational materials are at a 5th to 6th grade readability level.
  - Select content appropriate to learning objectives and allotted time frame.
  - Select an evaluation method that will provide feedback regarding achievement of short-term learning objectives, and long-term impact on behavior.
- Implement the education program. Ensure an environment that is conducive to learning (minimal distractions, favorable to interaction, learner comfort, readability).
- Evaluate the achievement of learning objectives and the effectiveness of instruction.

# *Epidemiology*

Epidemiology is the study of health-related trends in populations for the purposes of disease prevention, health maintenance, and health protection.

- Nurses use epidemiological principles to provide health interventions to targeted groups.
- Epidemiological calculations provide numerical information about the impact of disease and death on populations and aggregates.
- The epidemiological process is a systematic method of targeting a specific health need with the goal of improving health. Epidemiology provides a broad understanding of the spread, transmission, and incidence of disease and injury. This information is an important component of community assessment and program planning.
- Community health nurses are in the unique position of being able to identify cases and recognize patterns of disease, eliminate barriers to disease control, and provide education and counseling targeted at a disease condition or specific risk factors. Qᴏı

## EPIDEMIOLOGICAL TRIANGLE (1.3)

Epidemiology involves the study of the relationships among an agent, host, and environment (known as the epidemiological triangle). Their interaction determines the development and cessation of communicable diseases, as they form a web of causality, which increases or decreases the risk for disease.

- **The agent** is the physical, infectious, or chemical factor that causes the disease.
- **The host** is the living being that an agent or the environment influences.
- **The environment** is the setting or surrounding that sustains the host.

AGENT
HOST
ENVIRONMENT.

new/existing ÷ population × 1000.

## EPIDEMIOLOGICAL CALCULATIONS

Epidemiology relies on statistical evidence to determine the rate of spread of disease and the proportion of people affected. It also is used to evaluate the effectiveness of disease prevention and health promotion activities and to determine the extent to which goals are met.

## INCIDENCE AND PREVALENCE RATES

Incidence and prevalence rates are used to measure the existence of a particular disease, and allow the nurse to compare the rate of disease in one population to another, even though there can be different numbers of people in a given population.

> **Incidence:** Number of new cases in the population at a specific time ÷ population total x 1,000 = _____ per 1,000

> **Prevalence:** Number of existing cases in the population at a specific time ÷ population total x 1,000 = _____ per 1,000

## 1.3 Epidemiological triangle

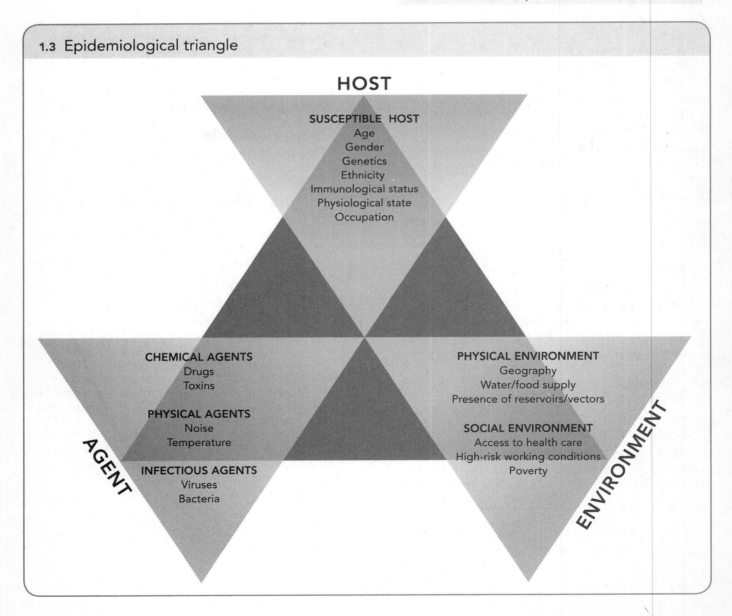

HOST

SUSCEPTIBLE HOST
Age
Gender
Genetics
Ethnicity
Immunological status
Physiological state
Occupation

CHEMICAL AGENTS
Drugs
Toxins

PHYSICAL AGENTS
Noise
Temperature

INFECTIOUS AGENTS
Viruses
Bacteria

PHYSICAL ENVIRONMENT
Geography
Water/food supply
Presence of reservoirs/vectors

SOCIAL ENVIRONMENT
Access to health care
High-risk working conditions
Poverty

AGENT

ENVIRONMENT

## MORTALITY RATES

Mortality rates provide information about cause of death. Public health workers can examine overall death rates (**crude mortality rate**), deaths from specific causes (**cause-specific rate**, **case fatality rate**), or deaths at specific times across the lifespan (**infant mortality ratio**, **age-specific rate**).

> **Crude mortality rate:** Number of deaths ÷ population total x 1,000 = _____ per 1,000

> **Infant mortality rate:** Number of infant deaths before 1 year of age in a year ÷ numbers of live births in the same year x 1,000 = _____ per 1,000

## ATTACK RATE

A disease or condition is endemic when there is a moderate, ongoing occurrence in a given location.

**Epidemic:** Occurs when the rate of disease exceeds the usual (endemic) level of the condition in a defined population.

**Pandemic:** Condition occurs when an epidemic occurs in multiple countries or continents.

> **Attack rate:** Number of people exposed to a specific agent who develop the disease ÷ total number of people exposed

## THE EPIDEMIOLOGICAL PROCESS

**Determine the nature, extent, and possible significance of the problem.** During this phase of the process, the nurse collects information from as many sources as possible. This information is then used to determine the scope of the problem.

**Using the gathered data, formulate a possible theory.** At this time, the nurse projects and explores the possible explanations.

**Gather information from a variety of sources in order to narrow down the possibilities.** The nurse assesses all possible sites for amassing information related to the disease process. The nurse evaluates the plausibility of the proposed hypothesis.

**Make the plan.** In this phase of the process, the nurse focuses on breaking the cycle of disease. The nurse should identify and consider all factors influencing the spread of the disease. The nurse establishes priorities to break the chain of transmission and to control the spread of the disease.

**Put the plan into action.** Using all available means, the nurse puts the plan for controlling the disease into action.

**Evaluate the plan.** The nurse gathers pertinent information to determine the success of the plan. Using this plan, the nurse evaluates the success in prevention of the spread of the disease.

**Report and follow up.** The nurse synthesizes evaluation data into a format that is understandable. Then the nurse evaluates successes and failures and bases follow-up on the evaluation information.

# Health promotion and disease prevention

- National health goals guide nurses in developing health promotion strategies to improve individual and community health.
- Community health nurses participate in three levels of prevention: primary, secondary, and tertiary.

## HEALTH PROMOTION

- National health goals are derived from scientific data and trends collected during the prior decade. These goals are based on those issues that are considered major risks to the health and wellness of the United States' population. Q**EBP**
  - ○ *Healthy People* was initiated in 1979, and every 10 years, publishes the national health objectives that serve as a guide for promoting health and preventing disease.
  - ○ *Healthy People* is coordinated by the U.S. Department of Health and Human Services, along with other federal agencies, and transitioned to *Healthy People 2020* in January 2010.
- *Healthy People* serves as a measure for quality of health. The national health goals guide the nurse in developing health promotion strategies to improve individual and community health.
- *Healthy People* initiatives have shown that implementing health promotion and disease prevention strategies leads to decreased expense for healthcare and improves the length of the client's lifespan.
- The community health nurse actively helps people to change their lifestyles in order to move toward a state of optimal health (physical and psychosocial).
- Preventive services include health education and counseling based on scientific evidence, immunizations, taking preventive medication, lifestyle changes and other actions that aim to prevent a potential disease or disability.
- The community health nurse provides preventive services in multiple community settings.
- The community health nurse is often responsible for planning and implementing screening programs for at-risk populations.
- Successful screening programs provide accurate, reliable results, can be inexpensively and quickly administered to large groups, and produce few if any adverse effects.
- The nurse should evaluate a potential screening method to determine whether it can be used consistently (reliability), it demonstrates accuracy of measurement (validity), and how effective it is at identifying an individual with a particular condition (predictive value).

# DISEASE PREVENTION

## Primary prevention

Prevention of the initial occurrence of disease or injury
- Nutrition education
- Family planning and sex education
- Smoking cessation education
- Communicable disease prevention education
- Education about health and hygiene issues to specific groups (day care workers, restaurant workers)
- Safety education (seat belt use, helmet use)
- Prenatal classes
- Providing immunizations
- Advocating for access to health care, healthy environments

## Secondary prevention

Early detection and treatment of disease with the goal of limiting severity and adverse effects
- Community assessments
- Disease surveillance (communicable diseases)
- Screenings
- Cancer (breast, cervical, testicular, prostate, colorectal)
- Diabetes mellitus
- Hypertension
- Hypercholesterolemia
- Sensory impairments
- Tuberculosis
- Lead exposure
- Genetic disorders/metabolic deficiencies in newborns
- Control of outbreaks of communicable diseases

## Tertiary prevention

- Maximization of recovery after an injury or illness (rehabilitation)
- Nutrition counseling for management of Crohn's disease
- Exercise rehabilitation
- Case management (chronic illness, mental illness)
- Physical and occupational therapy
- Support groups
- Exercise for a client who has hypertension (individual)

# Application Exercises

1. A nurse manager at a community agency is developing an orientation program for newly hired nurses. When discussing the differences between community-based and community-oriented nursing, the nurse should include which of the following situations as an example of community-based nursing? (Select all that apply.)

   A. A home health nurse performing wound care for a client who is immobile ●

   B. An occupational health nurse providing classes on body mechanics at a local industrial plant

   C. A school nurse teaching a student who has asthma about medications ●

   D. A parish nurse teaching a class on low-sodium cooking techniques

   E. A mental health nurse discussing stress management techniques with a support group

2. A nurse is advocating for local leaders to place a newly approved community health clinic in an area of the city that has fewer resources than other areas. The nurse is advocating for the leaders to uphold which of the following ethical principles?

   A. Distributive justice ●

   B. Fidelity

   C. Respect for autonomy

   D. Veracity

3. A nurse is preparing an education program on disease transmission for employees at a local day care facility. When discussing the epidemiological triangle, the nurse should include which of the following factors as agents? (Select all that apply.)

   A. Resource availability

   B. Ethnicity

   C. Toxins ●

   D. Bacteria ●

   E. Altered immunity

4. A nurse is developing a community health education program for a group of clients who have a new diagnosis of diabetes mellitus. Which of the following learning strategies should the nurse include for clients who are auditory learners?

   A. Showing informational videos ●

   B. Providing equipment to practice hands-on skills

   C. Supplying outlines for note-taking

   D. Facilitating small group discussions ●

5. A community health nurse is implementing health programs with several populations in the local area. In which of the following situations is the nurse using primary prevention?

   A. Performing a home safety check at a client's home

   B. Teaching healthy nutrition to clients who have hypertension

   C. Providing influenza immunizations to employees at a local preschool ●

   D. Implementing a program to notify individuals exposed to a communicable disease

---

**PRACTICE  Active Learning Scenario**

A school nurse is planning prevention activities for students. Use the ATI Active Learning Template: Basic Concept to complete this item.

**RELATED CONTENT**
- Define primary prevention.
- Define secondary prevention.
- Define tertiary prevention.

**NURSING INTERVENTIONS**
- Include two primary prevention activities the nurse should plan.
- Include two secondary prevention activities the nurse should plan.
- Include two tertiary prevention activities the nurse should plan.

# Application Exercises Key

1. A. **CORRECT:** The nurse should include wound care to an individual in the home as an example of community-based nursing, which involves management of acute and chronic conditions in a community setting.

B. The nurse should include teaching a class in the occupational setting as an example of community-oriented nursing, which involves health care of individuals, families and groups to improve the collective health of the community.

C. **CORRECT:** The nurse should include teaching a single student in the school setting as an example of community-based nursing, which involves management of acute and chronic conditions in a community setting.

D. The nurse should include teaching a class to members of a faith community as an example of community-oriented nursing, which involves health care of individuals, families and groups to improve the collective health of the community.

E. The nurse should include discussion with a group in the mental health setting as an example of community-oriented nursing, which involves health care of individuals, families and groups to improve the collective health of the community.

Ⓝ *NCLEX® Connection: Health Promotion and Maintenance, Health Promotion/Disease Prevention*

2. A. **CORRECT:** The nurse is advocating for the leaders to uphold the ethical principle of distributive justice, which is the fair distribution of benefits and burden in society.

B. The nurse is not advocating for the leaders to uphold the ethical principle of fidelity, which involves keeping commitments and following through with promises.

C. The nurse is not advocating for the leaders to uphold the ethical principle of respect for autonomy, which is supporting the rights of individuals to determine and pursue personal health care goals.

D. The nurse is not advocating for the leaders to uphold the ethical principle of veracity, which is the concept of telling the truth.

Ⓝ *NCLEX® Connection: Management of Care, Ethical Practice*

3. A. The nurse should include resource availability as an environmental factor when discussing the epidemiological triangle.

B. The nurse should include ethnicity as a host factor when discussing the epidemiological triangle.

C. **CORRECT:** The nurse should include toxins as an agent when discussing the epidemiological triangle.

D. **CORRECT:** The nurse should include bacteria as an agent when discussing the epidemiological triangle.

E. The nurse should include altered immunity as a host factor when discussing the epidemiological triangle.

Ⓝ *NCLEX® Connection: Safety and Infection Control, Standard Precautions/Transmission–Based Precautions/Surgical Asepsis*

4. A. The nurse should show informational videos as an appropriate learning strategy for clients who are visual learners.

B. The nurse should provide equipment to practice hands-on skills as an appropriate learning strategy for clients who are tactile-kinesthetic learners.

C. The nurse should supply outlines for note-taking as an appropriate learning strategy for clients who are visual learners.

D. **CORRECT:** Facilitating small group discussions provides an opportunity for clients who are auditory learners to learn as they listen to information. This is an appropriate strategy for the nurse to include for this group.

Ⓝ *NCLEX® Connection: Health Promotion and Maintenance, Health Promotion/Disease Prevention*

5. A. The nurse is using secondary prevention when performing a home safety check.

B. The nurse is using tertiary prevention when teaching healthy nutrition to clients who have hypertension.

C. **CORRECT:** The nurse is using primary prevention when providing influenza immunizations to employees at a local preschool because the goal is to prevent the occurrence of disease or injury.

D. The nurse is using secondary prevention when implementing a program to notify individuals exposed to a communicable disease.

Ⓝ *NCLEX® Connection: Health Promotion and Maintenance, Health Promotion/Disease Prevention*

## PRACTICE Answer

*Using the ATI Active Learning Template: Basic Concept*

### RELATED CONTENT

Primary prevention: Strategies that prevent the initial occurrence of disease or injury

Secondary prevention: Strategies that lead to early detection and treatment of disease with the goal of limiting severity and adverse effects

Tertiary prevention: Strategies that maximize recovery after an injury or illness

### NURSING INTERVENTIONS

Primary prevention activities
- Teaching healthy heart curriculum (nutrition, exercise, not smoking)
- Educating about dental health
- Discussing safety (seat belts, bicycle helmets, stranger safety)
- Administering immunizations
- Teaching about communicable disease transmission
- Providing sex education
- Advocating for safe playground equipment
- Providing substance use prevention education

Secondary prevention activities
- Performing tuberculin skin tests
- Performing routine checks for pediculosis
- Taking measures to control communicable disease outbreaks
- Screening for lead exposure
- Implementing scoliosis screenings
- Identifying students at risk for suicide or self-harm
- Performing vision and hearing screenings
- Measuring heights and weights
- Identifying indicators of child abuse or neglect

Tertiary prevention activities
- Teaching about allergic triggers for students who have asthma
- Administering medications to treat chronic conditions (asthma, attention deficit hyperactivity disorder, seizure disorders)
- Monitoring glucose levels and administering insulin to students who have diabetes mellitus
- Discussing and planning for nutritional needs of students who have cystic fibrosis
- Developing communication methods for students who have autism spectrum disorders

Ⓝ *NCLEX® Connection: Health Promotion and Maintenance, Health Promotion/Disease Prevention*

# NCLEX® Connections

When reviewing the following chapter, keep in mind the relevant topics and tasks of the NCLEX outline, in particular:

## Client Needs: Safety and Infection Control

**ACCIDENT/ERROR/INJURY PREVENTION:** Protect client from injury.

**HOME SAFETY:** Evaluate client care environment for fire/environmental hazard.

## Client Needs: Health Promotion and Maintenance

**DEVELOPMENTAL STAGES AND TRANSITIONS:** Recognize cultural and religious influences that may impact family functioning.

**HEALTH SCREENING:** Perform health history/ health and risk assessments.

**LIFESTYLE CHOICES:** Evaluate client alternative or homeopathic health care practices.

## Client Needs: Psychosocial Integrity

**CULTURAL AWARENESS/CULTURAL INFLUENCES ON HEALTH:** Evaluate and document how client language needs were met.

**STRESS MANAGEMENT:** Implement measures to reduce environmental stressors.

# Factors Influencing Community Health

Social determinants of health are factors that affect individual health. These are divided into five categories: neighborhood and built environment, social and community context, economic stability, health and healthcare, and education.

The family unit plays an important role in health. Family beliefs, cultural values, and environment can positively or negatively influence an individual's health. Genetic traits can affect family members' susceptibility to disease.

Culture is the beliefs, values, attitudes, and behaviors shared by a group of people and transmitted from generation to generation.

Environmental health refers to the influence of environmental conditions on the development of disease or injury.

Access to health care is impacted by the availability of services in a community, as well as individual, family, and community circumstances.

Nurses use data about genetics, family illnesses, the environment, and lifestyle to identify patterns of disease among family members, and to prevent and treat disease.

NEIGHBORHOOD and BUILT ENVIRONMENT.
.SOCIAL and COMMUNITY CONTEXT.
.ECONOMIC STABILITY.
.HEALTH and HEALTHCARE.
.EDUCATION.

five categories that affect human health.

## Cultural care

- The Office of Minority Health has requirements for culturally and linguistically appropriate services (CLAS). CLAS standards promote development of a healthcare workforce that can respond effectively to the needs of a diverse client population.
- CLAS standards include providing language assistance and information to a client in his preferred language throughout the delivery of health care.
- CLAS standards promote ongoing improvement and accountability for culturally appropriate care.
- Congruency between culture and health care is essential to the well-being of the client. The link between health beliefs and practices is greatly influenced by an individual's culture.
- It is important to assess cultural beliefs and practices when developing a plan of care. Qpcc
  - Community health nurses need to consider that there are variations within each culture.
  - Community health nurses should consider the uniqueness of each client.
  - Community health nurses should be familiar with cultures represented in the local community.

**Acculturation:** Acculturation is the process of merging with or adopting the traits of a different culture. Adapting to a new culture requires changes in daily living practices. These changes relate to language, education, work, recreation, social experiences, and the health care system.

**Cultural awareness:** Cultural awareness includes self-awareness of one's own cultural background, biases, and differences. Culturally aware nurses are:
- More likely to explore cultural variations among clients.
- Better able to understand how personal beliefs impact client care.
- Able to recognize that the meaning of health differs with each culture.

**Cultural needs:** Cultural needs of the client are as important as physical and psychological needs. The nurse should avoid imposing personal cultural values on the client, as well as ethnocentrism and stereotyping in the provision of care.

**Cultural competence:** Cultural competence involves respecting personal dignity and preferences, as well as acknowledging cultural differences.
- The provision of culturally competent care requires nurses to be responsive to the needs of clients from different cultures. Culturally competent care is guided by four dimensions.
  - **Cultural preservation:** Allowing preservation of the client's traditional values.
  - **Cultural accommodation:** Supporting and facilitating the client's use of cultural practices that are beneficial to the client's health.
  - **Cultural repatterning:** Assisting the client to modify cultural practices that are not beneficial to the client's health.
  - **Cultural brokering:** Advocating, mediating, negotiating, and intervening between the client's culture and health care culture on behalf of the client.
- Nurse leaders can use cultural competency in creating and working with a diverse workforce that can meet the needs of a diverse client population.

# CULTURAL ASSESSMENT

A cultural assessment provides information to the health care provider about the effect of culture on communication, space and physical contact, time, social organization, and environmental control factors.

## Environmental control

- Indicates the belief in how the environment affects the individual.
- Individuals who believe that the environment can be mastered to affect health status will actively engage in health promotion, disease prevention, and treatment.
- Individuals who feel that their outcome is predetermined and they cannot affect it are not as likely to engage in health-related behaviors.
- Individuals who believe in harmony with the environment are more likely to use alternative medicine and spirituality to promote balance in health status.

## Time orientation

- Describes whether an individual places more value on the past, the present or the future.
- Individuals who focus on the past or present can have little interest in health promotion behaviors, which are described as having benefit in the future.

## Social organization

- Describes the significance of individual members of a family or the family as a whole.
- A single family member who is not the client might be the decision maker in a family; an individual might forgo her own health care needs for the sake of the good of the family.

## Health beliefs and practices

Vary among cultures. Whatever an individual believes is the cause of impaired health will affect actions the individual will take to treat or prevent disease.

- **Biomedical beliefs** about illness focus on identifying a cause for every effect on the body; that the body functions like a machine. This is the basis for the United States health system and is science-based.
- **Naturalistic beliefs** about illness relate the individual as a part of nature or creation. An imbalance in nature is believed to cause disease. This is the basis of Eastern or Chinese medicine. Several other cultures, such as the Mexican culture, follow the hot-cold theory of balance in relation to health and illness that accompanies this belief framework.
- **Magico-religious beliefs** about illness link health to supernatural forces, or good and evil. This includes belief in faith healing used by some Christian religions, or voodoo and witchcraft practices used in Caribbean nations.

## Biological variations in health

Can be linked to genetic ties from biological relatives.

# CULTURAL ASSESSMENT PARAMETERS

- Ethnic background
- Religious preferences
- Family structure
- Language and literacy needs
- Communication needs
- Education
- Cultural values
- Food patterns
- Health practices
- Use of folk or spiritual healers and alternative healing techniques

## STEPS OF DATA COLLECTION

- The first step of the cultural assessment is collection of self-identifying data about the client's ethnic background, religious preference, family structure, food patterns, and health practices.
- Next, the nurse should pose questions that address the client's perceptions of his health needs.
- The final step of the data collection process is identification of how cultural factors can affect the effectiveness of nursing interventions.

## USING AN INTERPRETER

- The nurse should use an interpreter when it is difficult for a nurse or client to understand the other's language.
- Interpreters should have knowledge of health-related terminology.
- The use of family members as interpreters is not advisable because clients might need privacy in discussing sensitive matters. Family members can lack objectivity when relaying information to or from the client, and the family member can have difficulty understanding medical terminology.
- The nurse should consider client preferences when selecting the age and gender of an interpreter.
- Interpreters should not be from the same community as the client.
- Differences in socioeconomic status, religious affiliation, educational level, and spoken dialectic can result in translation barriers.
- Federal government mandates require agencies to have a plan that will improve access to federal health care programs for individuals who have limited English proficiency.

## CULTURAL COMPETENCE SELF-ASSESSMENT

- Am I aware of my culture and views about other cultures?
- Am I able to perform a culturally sensitive assessment?
- Do I have the knowledge necessary to develop culturally appropriate nursing interventions?
- What is my goal in learning about diverse populations?

## CONVEYING CULTURAL SENSITIVITY

- Address clients by their last names, unless the client gives the nurse permission to use other names.
- Introduce yourself by name and explain your position.
- Be authentic and honest about what is known or not known about a client's culture.
- Use culturally sensitive language.
- Find out what clients know about their health problems and treatments, and assess cultural congruence.
- Incorporate clients' preferences and practices into care when possible.
- Do not make assumptions about clients.
- Encourage clients to ask about anything that they might not understand.
- Respect clients' values, beliefs, and practices.
- Show respect for clients' support systems.
- Provide health teaching materials in the client's primary language and at the recommended readability level.

5-6 grade level.

# *Environmental health*

Environmental health relates to the quality of the air, land, water, and other surroundings to which people come into contact.

- Nurses identify environmental health risk, participate in research, and use advocacy to improve environmental quality.
- Nurses can contribute to environmental health by engaging in environmentally friendly practices and use of material, as well as providing information to the public about environmental health.
- Toxicology considers how exposure to chemicals can have negative effects on health. Nurses use toxicological information to understand the specific effects that environmental hazards have on populations at risk or following exposure. Data is available through the National Library of Medicine at www.nlm.nih.gov.

## ENVIRONMENTAL RISKS

**Toxins:** lead, pesticides, mercury, solvents, asbestos, and radon

**Air pollution:** carbon monoxide, particulate matter, ozone, lead, aerosols, nitrogen dioxide, sulfur dioxide, and tobacco smoke

**Water pollution:** wastes, erosion after mining or timbering, and run-off from chemicals added to the soil.

**Contamination:** food and food products with bacteria, pesticides, radiation, and medication (growth hormones or antibiotics)

## ROLES FOR NURSES

- Facilitate public participation in measures to improve the environment.
- Perform individual and population risk assessments.
- Implement risk communication.
- Conduct epidemiological investigations.
- Participate in policy development.

## ASSESSMENT

The "I PREPARE" mnemonic is one method of determining current and past environmental exposures. Qs

**I: Investigate** potential exposures

**P: Present work:** exposures, use of personal protective equipment, location of safety data sheets (SDS), hazardous materials brought home from work on clothing, trends

**R: Residence:** age of home, heating, recent remodeling, chemical storage, water

**E: Environmental concerns:** air, water, soil, industries in neighborhood, waste site or landfill nearby

**P: Past work:** exposures, farm work, military, volunteer, seasonal, length of work

**A: Activities:** hobbies, activities, gardening, fishing, hunting, soldering, melting, burning, eating, pesticides, alternative healing/medicines

**R: Referrals and resources:** Environmental Protection Agency, Agency for Toxic Substances & Disease Registry, Association of Occupational and Environmental Clinics, SDS, OSHA, local health department, environmental agency, poison control

**E: Educate:** risk reduction, prevention, follow-up

## KEY QUESTIONS FOR HEALTH HISTORY

- Housing: What is the physical condition, age or location of the residence?, Is it located near a school, day care, or work site? Are lighting, ventilation, and heating/cooling systems adequate?
- What are the occupations of household members (current and past, longest-held jobs)?
- Is tobacco smoke present?
- Are there any recent home remodeling activities, such as the installation of new carpet or furniture or refinishing of furniture?
- What hobbies are done in the home?
- Is there any other recent exposure to chemicals or radiation?
- Are pets present in the home, and are they healthy?
- Has there been any lead exposure in old paint, crafts, leaded pottery, or dishes?
- What is the source and quality of the drinking water?
- How is sewage and waste disposed of in the home?
- Are there pesticides used around the home or garden?
- Is there any water damage or evidence of mold or fungi?
- Where do children play? Is there any hazardous play equipment or toys?
- Does the surrounding neighborhood present any hazards with closeness to highways or small businesses, such as dry cleaning, photo processing, industry, or auto repair?

# NATIONAL HEALTH CARE GOALS

## REDUCTIONS

- Toxic air emissions
- Waterborne disease outbreaks
- Per capita domestic water use
- Blood lead levels in children
- Pesticide exposures requiring visits to health care facility
- Indoor allergen levels
- U.S. homes with lead-based paint or related hazards
- Exposure to chemicals and pollutants
- Risks posed by hazardous sites
- Number of new schools near highways
- Global burden of disease due to environmental concerns

## INCREASES

- Use of alternative modes of transportation for work
- Number of days that beaches are open and safe for swimming
- Recycling of municipal solid waste
- Testing for presence of lead-based paint in pre-1978 housing
- Monitoring for diseases or conditions caused by environmental hazards
- Homes with radon mitigation (those at-risk) and radon-reducing features
- Schools with policies/practices to promote health/safety
- Presence/use of information systems related to environmental health

*[handwritten left margin: only 1978 or before for lead based paint]*

# NURSING INTERVENTIONS

## PRIMARY PREVENTION

INDIVIDUAL: Educate individuals to reduce environmental hazards.

### COMMUNITY

- Educate groups to reduce environmental hazards.
- Advocate for safe air and water.
- Support programs for waste reduction and recycling.
- Advocate for waste reduction and effective waste management.

## SECONDARY PREVENTION

### INDIVIDUAL

- Survey for health conditions that can be related to environmental and occupational exposures.
- Obtain environmental health histories of individuals.
- Monitor workers for levels of chemical exposures at job sites.
- Screen children 6 months to 5 years old for blood lead levels.

### COMMUNITY

- Survey for health conditions that can be related to environmental and occupational exposures.
- Assess neighborhoods, schools, work sites, and the community for environmental hazards.

# TERTIARY PREVENTION

## INDIVIDUAL

- Refer homeowners to lead abatement resources.
- Educate clients who have asthma about environmental triggers.

## COMMUNITY

- Become active in consumer and health-related organizations and legislation related to environmental health issues.
- Support cleanup of toxic waste sites and removal of other hazards.

# *Global health*

- Health care delivery and health problems around the world affect the health of countries.
- Global health initiatives can be used to improve health status worldwide, and to promote equity in treatment.
- *Health for All in the 21st Century* (HFA21) outlines goals to promote productivity through adequate healthcare services around the globe.
- Examining the years of life lost from early death and disability provides information about the global burden of disease.

## INFLUENCES ON GLOBAL HEALTH

- Wars and political unrest
- Natural and man-made disasters
- Limited resources and structure in lesser-developed nations
- International travel (increases spread of disease)
- Sanitation practices
- Climate change
- Maternal health
- Nutrition

## GOALS FOR GLOBAL HEALTH

The United Nations created the Millennium Developmental Goals (MDGs) which called for more developed nations to contribute resources to improve conditions in lesser-developed countries, making global health a responsibility of nations around the world. The MDGs include the following. Qᵒⁱ

- Eradicating hunger and extreme poverty
- Making primary education available worldwide
- Promoting empowerment of women and gender equality
- Reducing child mortality
- Fostering maternal health
- Reducing malaria, HIV/AIDS, and other communicable diseases
- Promoting a sustainable environment
- Developing global partnerships

## NURSING INTERVENTIONS

- Support the development of health care roles in countries that lack health care professionals.
- Promote the benefits of nursing as a distinct profession in health promotion and disease prevention and reducing health care costs.
- Work with governments and other developers of policy to promote the rights of nurses.
- Foster programs that promote environmental sustainability ("go green" campaigns to preserve natural resources, recycling facilities).
- Act as mentors or consultants to address health of individuals and communities in other countries.

# *Access to health care*

- The goal of a primary health care system is to make health care available in close proximity to people who need it, and to ensure that it be comprehensive with flexible cost to accommodate the income variations of the individuals who use those services.
- Community health nurses must advocate for improved access to health care services.
- Community health nurses can help shift the focus of the health care system from acute treatment of disease to primary prevention measures, in order to decrease health care costs and promote equity.
- Community assessment includes evaluating the adequacy of health services within the community and the accessibility of those services by those needing access.
- It is important to identify barriers that community members, particularly vulnerable populations, encounter when accessing health services.

### BARRIERS TO HEALTH CARE
- Inadequate health care insurance
- Inability to pay for health care services
- Language barriers
- Cultural barriers
- Lack of health care providers in a community
- Geographic isolation
- Social isolation
- Lack of communication tools (e.g., telephones)
- Lack of personal or public transportation to health care facilities
- Inconvenient hours
- Attitudes of health care personnel toward clients of low socioeconomic status or those with different cultural/ethnic backgrounds
- Eligibility requirements for state/federal assistance programs

## ORGANIZATIONS AND FINANCING

Although providing health care is a human service, health care delivery is also a business, affected by economic influences. Good health status, in turn, positively affects the economy by increasing the individual's potential for productivity and wage-earning.

- **Microeconomic theory** examines individual preference and finances, and how those actions affect cost of care and resource distribution.
- **Macroeconomic theory** focuses on aggregate behaviors, economic growth, and employment.
- The cost associated with health care is a barrier to care for many. Some providers ration health care, and only offer services to individuals with certain coverage types.
- In the U.S., the government is involved in providing direct health care services, providing information and protection to the public, setting policies, and assisting providers and the public with finances.

## AFFORDABLE CARE ACT

- The Patient Protection and Affordable Care Act was created to help make health insurance affordable for all people and decrease the amount of federal spending on health care. It affects the way Medicare benefits are implemented and the way private insurance companies supply coverage.
- The full law is available through the U.S. Department of Health and Human Services website, www.hhs.gov.

### IMPORTANT ELEMENTS OF THE AFFORDABLE CARE ACT
- Extending eligibility for dependents to remain on parent's insurance until age 26.
- Prohibiting health plans from denying benefits for preexisting coverage to children under age 19.
- Banning lifetime limits on benefit coverage.
- Covering preventive care services.

## ORGANIZATIONS

The health care system in the U.S. is influenced by federal and private organizations (insurers, employers), as well as global health organizations.

### *International health organizations*

**World Health Organization (WHO)**
- Provides daily information regarding the occurrence of internationally important diseases.
- Establishes world standards for antibiotics and vaccines.
- Primarily focuses on the health care workforce and education, environment, sanitation, infectious diseases, maternal and child health, and primary care.

## Federal health agencies

**Veterans Health Administration**
Finances health services for active and retired military persons and dependents (within the U.S. Department of Veterans Affairs).

**U.S. Department of Health & Human Services**
- Under the direction of the Secretary of Health
- Funded through federal taxes
- Consists of the following agencies.
  - **Administration for Children and Families (ACF)**
  - **Administration for Community Living (ACL)**
  - **Centers for Medicare and Medicaid Services (CMS):** Also administers the Health Insurance Portability and Accountability Act (HIPAA), disability insurance, Aid to Families with Dependent Children (AFDC), and Supplemental Security Income (SSI). **(2.1)**
  - **Agency for Healthcare Research and Quality (AHRQ):** Conducts research to improve the quality, affordability, and safety of healthcare services. Uses research data to publish clinical guidelines and recommendations for a variety of health conditions. Qᵒᴵ
  - **Centers for Disease Control and Prevention (CDC):** Works to prevent and control disease, injury, and disability both nationally and internationally.
  - **Agency for Toxic Substances and Disease Registry (ATSDR):** Strives to decrease harmful exposure and diseases linked to toxic substances.
  - **Food and Drug Administration (FDA):** Works to ensure food safety as well as the safety and effectiveness of medications.
  - **Health Resources and Service Administration (HRSA):** Includes the Division of Nursing, Division of Medicine and Dentistry, and the Division of Public Health and Interdisciplinary Education.
  - **Indian Health Service (IHS):** Promotes tribal health for American Indians and Alaskan Natives.
  - **National Institutes of Health (NIH):** Supports biomedical research and includes the National Institute of Nursing Research.
  - **Substance Abuse and Mental Health Services Administration (SAMHSA):** Promotes behavioral health and aims to reduce the negative effects of substance use and mental illness.

## State health agencies

**State departments of health:** Obtain funding from state legislature and federal public health agencies.
- Manages the **Women, Infants and Children (WIC)** program, which promotes nutrition for women, infants, and children up to age five who are of low socioeconomic status.
- Oversees **Children's Health Insurance Program (CHIP)**, which offers expanded health coverage to uninsured children whose families do not qualify for Medicaid.
- Establishes public health policies.
- Provides assistance/support for local health departments.
- Responsible for the administration of the Medicaid program.
- Reports notifiable communicable diseases within the state to the CDC.

**State boards of nursing**
- Development and oversight of the state's nurse practice act.
- Licensure of registered and licensed practical nurses.
- Oversight of the state's schools of nursing.

## Local health department

Receives funds from the state level to implement community level programs.
- The primary focus of a local health department is the health of its citizens.
- Local health departments offer various services and programs.
- Responsible for identifying and intervening to meet health needs of the local community.
- Work closely with local officials, businesses, and stakeholders.
- Report notifiable communicable diseases to state departments of health.
- Nurses at the community level typically function in the nursing roles of caregiver, advocate, case manager, referral source, counselor, educator, outreach worker, disease surveillance expert, community mobilizer and disaster responder.
- Funded through local taxes with support from federal and state funds.

---

### 2.1 Medicare and Medicaid at a glance

*Medicare* ~~OLDER THAN 65 OR ESKD.~~
Individuals must be older than 65 years and receiving Social Security, have been receiving disability benefits for 2 years, have amyotrophic lateral sclerosis and receive disability benefits, or have kidney failure and be on maintenance dialysis or had a kidney transplant to qualify for Medicare.

Part A (hospital care, home care, hospice, limited skilled nursing care)

Part B (health care provider services, outpatient care, home health, diagnostic services, physiotherapy, durable medical equipment, ambulance service, mental health, preventive services)

Part C (also known as the Medicare Advantage plan: is a combination of Part A and Part B and is provided through a private insurance company)

Part D (prescription medication coverage)

*Medicaid*
Medicaid provides health care coverage for individuals of low socioeconomic status and children, through the combined efforts of federal and state governments. Eligibility is based on household size and income, with priority given to children, pregnant women, and those who have a disability.

Medicaid provides inpatient and outpatient hospital care, laboratory and radiology services, home health care, vaccines for children, family planning, pregnancy-related care, and Early and Periodic Screening, Diagnosis, and Treatment (EPSDT) services for those younger than 21 years.

## Private funding

HEALTH INSURANCE

EMPLOYER BENEFITS

MANAGED CARE: is based on using a case management approach with a specific group of providers in an attempt to contain the cost of care.

- **Health maintenance organizations (HMOs):** Comprehensive care is provided to members by a set of designated providers.
- **Preferred provider organizations (PPOs):** Predetermined rates are set for services delivered to members; financial incentives are in place to promote use of PPO providers.
- **Medical savings accounts:** Untaxed money is put in an account for use for medical expenses.

## Self-pay

Individuals are responsible for payment of charges not covered by a third party. Some clinics offer sliding scale payment where the rate of payment is based on the individual income.

## NURSING INTERVENTIONS

- Use community assessment to identify barriers to adequate health care.
- Maintain awareness of healthcare standards and organizations that influence care delivery.
- Promote distributive justice in the use of health care resources.
- Understand the partnership and communication between local, state, and federal health entities. Qᴛᴄ
- Assist individuals and groups in obtaining adequate access to care, and work to promote equity in health care delivery.
- Maintain knowledge and skill related to economic principles, which can be applied to budgeting and funding of care.

# Application Exercises

1. A nurse is preparing an educational program on cultural perspectives in nursing. The nurse should include that which of the following factors are influenced by an individual's culture? (Select all that apply.)

   A. Nutritional practices
   B. Family structure
   C. Health care interactions
   D. Biological variations
   E. Views about illness

2. A nurse is caring for a client who is from a different culture than himself. When beginning the cultural assessment, which of the following actions should the nurse take first?

   A. Determine the client's perception of his current health status.
   B. Gather data about the client's cultural beliefs.
   C. Determine how the client's culture can affect the effectiveness of nursing actions.
   D. Gather information about previous client interactions with the health care system.

3. A nurse is using the I PREPARE mnemonic to assess a client's potential environmental exposures. Which of the following questions should the nurse ask when assessing for "A" in the mnemonic?

   A. "What do you like to do for fun?"
   B. "What year was your residence built?"
   C. "What jobs have you had in the past?"
   D. "What industries are near where you live?"

   *ACTIVITIES. "A.*

4. A nurse is reviewing information about the local health department to prepare for an interview. Which of the following services should the nurse expect the local health department to provide? (Select all that apply.)

   A. Managing the Women, Infants, and Children program
   B. Providing education to achieve community health goals
   C. Coordinating directives from state personnel
   D. Reporting communicable diseases to the CDC
   E. Licensing of registered nurses

5. A nurse is conducting health screenings at a statewide health fair and identifies several clients who require referral to a provider. Which of the following statements by a client indicates a barrier to accessing health care?

   A. "I don't drive, and my son is only available to take me places in the mornings."
   B. "I can't take off during the day, and the local after-hours clinic is no longer in operation."
   C. "Only one doctor in my town is a designated provider by my health maintenance organization."
   D. "I would like to schedule an appointment with the local doctor in my town who speaks Spanish and English."

---

**PRACTICE** Active Learning Scenario

A nurse is conducting an environmental health history during a postpartum home visit. Residents in the home include the mother, her partner, a 1-week-old infant, 2 year-old toddler, and 7-year-old child. Use the ATI Active Learning Template: Basic Concept to complete this item.

**UNDERLYING PRINCIPLES**
- Include two national health goals that relate to this family.
- Include two questions to ask as part of the environmental health history.

**NURSING INTERVENTIONS:** Include two primary and two secondary prevention interventions.

# Application Exercises Key

1. A. **CORRECT:** Culture is the beliefs, values, attitudes, and behaviors shared by a group of people and transmitted from generation to generation. The nurse should understand that nutritional practices are influenced by an individual's culture.

   B. **CORRECT:** Culture is the beliefs, values, attitudes, and behaviors shared by a group of people and transmitted from generation to generation. The nurse should understand that family structure is influenced by an individual's culture.

   C. **CORRECT:** Culture is the beliefs, values, attitudes, and behaviors shared by a group of people and transmitted from generation to generation. The nurse should understand that health care interactions are influenced by an individual's culture.

   D. Biological variations are physical, biological and physiological differences between races, and are not influenced by the beliefs, values, and attitudes of an individual.

   E. **CORRECT:** Culture is the beliefs, values, attitudes, and behaviors shared by a group of people and transmitted from generation to generation. The nurse should understand that views about illness are influenced by an individual's culture.

   Ⓝ *NCLEX® Connection: Psychosocial Integrity, Cultural Awareness/Cultural Influences on Health*

2. A. It is important for the nurse to determine the client's perception of his current health status. However, when conducting a cultural assessment, the nurse should perform a different action first.

   B. **CORRECT:** The nurse's first action when beginning a cultural assessment is to collect self-identifying data about the client, including specific information about how the client's cultural beliefs influence family structure, food patterns, religious preferences, and health practices.

   C. While it is important for the nurse to determine how the client's culture can affect the effectiveness of nursing actions, the nurse must gather other information first.

   D. It is important for the nurse to gather information about previous client interactions with the health care system. However, when conducting a cultural assessment, the nurse should perform a different action first.

   Ⓝ *NCLEX® Connection: Psychosocial Integrity, Cultural Awareness/Cultural Influences on Health*

3. A. **CORRECT:** The "A" in I-PREPARE mnemonic represents activities. The nurse should ask this question to determine hobbies and interests that might cause harm or expose the client to harmful substances.

   B. The nurse should ask this question to assess the first "R," which represents residence in the mnemonic.

   C. The nurse should ask this question to assess the second "P," which represents past work in the mnemonic.

   D. The nurse should ask this question to assess the first "E," which represents environmental concerns in the mnemonic.

   Ⓝ *NCLEX® Connection: Safety and Infection Control, Accident/Error/Injury Prevention*

4. A. The nurse should expect state departments of health to manage the Women, Infants, and Children (WIC) program.

   B. **CORRECT:** Providing education to achieve community health goals is a component of identifying and intervening to meet health needs of the local community, which is a responsibility of local health departments.

   C. **CORRECT:** Funding for local health departments comes from local, state, and federal monies. Local health departments are responsible for coordinating directives issued from the state level.

   D. The nurse should expect state departments of health to report communicable diseases to the CDC. Local health departments report communicable diseases to the state department of health.

   E. The nurse should expect state boards of nursing to supervise licensure of registered nurses.

   Ⓝ *NCLEX® Connection: Management of Care, Case Management*

5. A. Because the client has some form of transportation to the provider, this statement does not represent a barrier to accessing health care. The nurse should instruct the client to schedule a follow-up appointment when the family member is available to drive.

   B. **CORRECT:** Inconvenient hours make scheduling a follow-up appointment challenging, and indicates a barrier to accessing health care for this client.

   C. Because this client has an available provider, even though it is the only option, this statement does not represent a barrier to accessing health care. The nurse should instruct the client to schedule a follow-up appointment with this provider.

   D. The presence of a provider who is bilingual represents increased access to health care because it increases accessibility for clients who might speak a different language.

   Ⓝ *NCLEX® Connection: Health Promotion and Maintenance, Health Promotion/Disease Prevention*

---

## PRACTICE Answer

*Using the ATI Active Learning Template: Basic Concept*

### UNDERLYING PRINCIPLES

National health goals
- Reduction in per capita domestic water usage
- Reduction in blood lead levels in children
- Reduction in indoor allergens
- Reduction in the number of new schools near highways
- Increase in schools with policies/practices to promote health and safety

Environmental health history
- What year was your home built?
- What is your and your partner's current occupation?
- What recreational activities do your family participate in?
- Are there any industries or hazardous waste sites nearby?
- Where does your drinking water come from?

### NURSING INTERVENTIONS

Primary prevention
- Educate the mother and her partner about home safety for children.
- Teach the mother and her partner about potential sources of lead in the home.

Secondary prevention
- Screen children for lead exposure.
- Screen for potential chemical exposure of the mother and her partner at their places of employment.

Ⓝ *NCLEX® Connection: Safety and Infection Control, Accident/Error/Injury Prevention*

When reviewing the following chapter, keep in mind the relevant topics and tasks of the NCLEX outline, in particular:

## Client Needs: Management of Care

**COLLABORATION WITH INTERPROFESSIONAL TEAM:** Collaborate with interprofessional members when providing client care.

**CONTINUITY OF CARE:** Follow up on unresolved issues regarding client care.

**PERFORMANCE IMPROVEMENT (QUALITY IMPROVEMENT):** Evaluate the impact of performance improvement measures on client care and resource utilization.

## Client Needs: Health Promotion and Maintenance

**HEALTH PROMOTION/DISEASE PREVENTION:** Identify risk factors for disease/illness.

**HIGH RISK BEHAVIORS:** Assess client lifestyle practice risks that may impact health.

## Client Needs: Psychosocial Integrity

**BEHAVIORAL INTERVENTIONS:** Participate in group sessions.

**CULTURAL AWARENESS/CULTURAL INFLUENCES ON HEALTH:** Incorporate client cultural practice and beliefs when planning and providing care.

**THERAPEUTIC ENVIRONMENT:** Identify external factors that may interfere with client recovery.

Formulate Question(s).
Review Literature.
Design Study.
Analyze Findings.

Tertiary care is ↓ in rural areas.

Tdap can be given to pregnant women
b/w 27-36 weeks.

# Community Health Program Planning

The role of the community health nurse in community health program planning and evaluation is a collaborative leadership role. The desired outcome is the improved health of the community through the role and functions of the community health nurse.

The nurse can use program planning to promote healthy communities, in which community members partner with the nurse to address significant health issues.

Community health program planning should reflect the priorities set as a result of analysis of community assessment data. Priorities are established based on the extent of the problem (community members' perception of health needs, percent of population affected by the problem), the relevance of the problem to the public (degree of risk, economic loss), and the estimated effect of intervention (improvement of health outcome, adverse effects).

## ECOLOGICAL MODEL

An ecological model for population health can be used as a guide to examine the determinants of health for a population, and for targeting interventions to multiple factors that affect health. It includes the following components.
- Individual traits (age; gender; biological, mental, and behavioral factors)
- Social, family, and community relationships
- Occupational and home environments
- Overall conditions created by local, state, national, and worldwide forces and trends

## COMMUNITY ASSESSMENT: INDIVIDUAL, FAMILY, AGGREGATES

- Community assessment is a comprehensive approach that emphasizes the community as a client, with the goal of providing benefit to the people of the area as a whole, rather than to individuals. Qpcc
- Community assessment and diagnosis are the foundation for community-specific program planning.
- Using the nursing process, nurses can determine health needs within the community and assist in developing and implementing strategies to meet those needs. In doing this, it is necessary to expand the assessment, diagnosis, planning, intervention, and evaluation efforts from the individual to the community or aggregate level.

## COMMUNITY HEALTH NURSE ROLES

The community health nurse is a key player in assessing the needs of the community.
- Interacting and establishing contracts with community partners serving the community at large
- Witnessing the interaction between community programs and the response of the client to the services
- Identifying future services based upon the visible needs of community members and population groups

## FACTORS TO CONSIDER

When determining the health of a community

**Status:** Epidemiological data, client satisfaction, mental health, crime rates

**Structure:** Presence of health care facilities, service types and patterns of use, demographic data

**Process:** Relationships, communication, commitment to and participation in health

## COMMUNITY ASSESSMENT COMPONENTS

### People

**Demographic:** Distribution, mobility, density, census data

**Biological factors:** Health and disease status, genetics, race, age, gender, causes of death

**Social factors:** Occupation, activities, marital status, education, income, crime rates, recreation, industry

**Cultural factors:** Ethnohistory, hierarchy and roles, language, religion and spirituality, values, customs, norms

## Place or environment

**Physical factors:** Geography, terrain, type of community, location of health services, housing, animal control

**Environmental factors:** Geography, climate, flora, fauna, topography, toxic substances, vectors, pollutants

## Social systems

- Health systems
- Economic systems/factors
- Education systems
- Religious systems
- Welfare systems
- Political systems
- Recreation systems/factors
- Legal systems
- Communication systems/factors
- Transportation systems
- Resources and services

# DATA COLLECTION

Data collection is a critical community health nursing function. To best identify the health needs of the local community, it is essential to combine several methods of data collection. Relying on only one or two key pieces can result in an incomplete assessment.

## Informant interviews

Direct discussion with community members for the purpose of obtaining ideas and opinions from key informants

STRENGTHS
- Minimal cost
- Participants serving as future supporters
- Offers insight into beliefs and attitudes of community members
- Reading/writing of participants not required
- Personal interaction can elicit more detailed responses

LIMITATIONS
- Built-in bias
- Meeting time and place

## Community forum

Open public meeting

STRENGTHS
- Opportunity for community input
- Minimal cost

LIMITATIONS
- Difficulty finding a convenient time and place
- Potential to drift from the issue
- Challenging to get adequate participation
- Possibility that a less vocal person can be reluctant to speak

## Secondary data

Use of existing data (death, birth statistics; census data; mortality, morbidity data; health records; minutes from meetings; prior health surveys) to assess problem

The nurse must evaluate the reliability of secondary data obtained from the Web. Generally, websites with .edu, .org, and .gov URLs present reliable information. Qu

STRENGTHS
- Database of prior concerns/needs of population
- Ability to trend health issues over time

LIMITATIONS
- Possibility that data might not represent current situation
- Can be time-consuming

## Participant observation

Observation of formal or informal community activities

STRENGTHS: Indication of community priorities, environmental profile, and identification of power structures

LIMITATIONS
- Bias
- Time-consuming
- Inability to ask questions of participants

## Focus groups

Directed talk with a representative sample

STRENGTHS
- Possibility of participants being potential supporters
- Provides insight into community support
- Reading/writing of participants not required

LIMITATIONS
- Possible discussion of irrelevant issues
- Challenging to get participants
- Requires strong facilitator
- Difficult to ensure that sample is truly representative of the overall community
- Time-consuming to transcribe discussion

## Surveys

Specific questions asked in a written format

STRENGTHS
- Data collected on client population and problems
- Random sampling
- Available as written or online format
- Contact with participants not required

LIMITATIONS
- Low response rate
- Expensive
- Time-consuming
- Possibility of collection of superficial data
- Requires reading/writing abilities of participants

## Windshield survey

Descriptive approach that assesses several community components by driving through a community

STRENGTHS: Provides a descriptive overview of a community

LIMITATIONS
- Need for a driver so the nurse can visualize and document the community elements
- Can be time-consuming
- Results based only on visualization and does not include input from community members

SURVEY COMPONENTS
- **People**
  - Who is on the street?
  - What is their general appearance (age, dress, well-nourished, obese, frail, unkempt)?
  - What are they doing?
  - What is the origin, ethnicity, or race of the people?
  - How are the different groups (subgroups) residentially located?
  - Is there any evidence of substance use, violence, disease, mental illness?
  - Are there any animals or pets in the community?
- **Place**
  - Boundaries
    - Where is the community located?
    - What are its boundaries?
    - Are there natural boundaries?
    - Are there man-made boundaries?
  - Location of health services
    - Where are the major health facilities located?
    - What health care facilities are necessary for the community but are not within the community?
  - Natural environment
    - Are there geographic features that can harm the community?
    - Are there plants or animals that could harm or threaten the health of the community?
  - Man-made environment
    - What industries are within the communities?
    - Could the environment or industry pose a threat to the health of community workers or the community itself?
    - Is there easy access to health care facilities?
    - Are the roads adequate and marked well?
    - What types of employment exist? Manufacturing? Retail? Small business? Military installation?
    - Are there grocery stores which provide fresh produce, or is this a "food desert"?
    - Where is garbage disposed? Is there evidence of trash, abandoned cars or houses?
- **Housing**
  - Is the housing of acceptable quality?
  - How old are the homes?
  - Are there single or multifamily dwellings?
  - Is the housing in good repair or disrepair?
  - Is there vacant housing?

- **Social systems**
  - Are there social services, clinics, hospitals, dentists, and health care providers available within the community?
  - Are there ample schools within the community? Are they in good repair or disrepair?
  - Are there parks or areas for recreation?
  - What places of worship are within the community?
  - What services are provided by local religious groups, schools, community centers, and activity or recreation centers?
  - Is there public transportation?
  - What grocery stores or other stores are within the community?
  - Is public protection evident (police, fire, emergency medical services, animal control)?

## ANALYSIS OF COMMUNITY ASSESSMENT DATA

- The community health nurse plays an active role in assessment, data interpretation, and problem identification. Steps in analysis of community assessment data include the following.
  - Gathering collected data into a composite database
  - Assessing completeness of data
  - Identifying and generating missing data
  - Synthesizing data and identifying themes
  - Identifying community needs and problems
  - Identifying community strengths and resources
- Problem analysis is completed for each identified problem. Frequently, work groups are formed to examine individual problems and develop solutions. Qᵒⁱ

## COMMUNITY HEALTH DIAGNOSES

- Problems identified by community assessments are often stated as community health diagnoses.
- Community nursing diagnoses incorporate information from the community assessment, general nursing knowledge, and epidemiological concepts (especially the concept of risk in a population).
- Community nursing diagnoses often are written in the following format.

**Risk of** [specific problem or risk in the community] **among** [the specific population that is affected by the problem or risk] **related to** [strengths and weaknesses in the community that influence the problem or risk].

**Risk of** low birth weight **among** adolescents who are pregnant in the downtown district **related to** low income, lack of availability of nutritious food, and tobacco use as evidenced by lack of secure housing, food bank use, increased rates of unemployment, and smoking among pregnant adolescents.

# COMMUNITY HEALTH PROGRAM PLANNING, DEVELOPMENT, AND MANAGEMENT

Nurses should consider literacy needs when developing interventions. An individual's ability to understand basic health information and make decisions, or health literacy, can affect the ability or desire to take action.

## Preplanning

Brainstorm ideas.
- Gain entry into community and establish trust.
- Obtain community awareness, support, and involvement.
- Coordinate collaborations that have similar interests in addressing identified problems.

## Assessment

Collect data about the community and its members.
- Complete a needs assessment and identify community strengths and weaknesses.
- Assess the availability of community resources.
- List potential sources for program funding (charitable giving, fund-raising, grants).
- Evaluate secondary health data.

## Diagnosis

Identify and prioritize health needs of the community.
- Analyze data to determine health needs.
- Work with community members, local health professionals and administrators to develop priorities and establish outcomes.
- In setting priorities among identified community problems, consider the following.
  - Community awareness of the problem
  - Community readiness to acknowledge and address the problem
  - Available expertise/fiscal resources
  - Severity of the problem
  - Amount of time needed for problem resolution

## Planning

Develop interventions to meet identified outcomes.
- Determine possible solutions to meet the health need.
- Compare the resources and interventions required for each solution, and select the best option.
- Establish goals and objectives for the selected solution.
  - Objectives are behaviorally stated, measurable, and include a target date for achievement.
- Select strategies/interventions to meet the objectives.
- Plan a logical sequence for interventions by establishing a timetable.
- Identify who will assume responsibility for each intervention. Qᵀᶜ
- Determine available and needed resources to implement interventions.
- Assess the personnel needed and any special training required for screening or providing education.
- Determine funding opportunities for needed interventions and develop a budget.
- Plan for program evaluation.

## Implementation

Carry out the plan.
- Initiate interventions to achieve goals and objectives according to program plan.
- Monitor the intervention process and the response of the community in terms of values, needs, and perceptions.

## Evaluation

Examine the success of the interventions.
- Evaluate strengths and weaknesses of the program.
- Determine achievement of desired outcomes.
- Examine the adequacy, efficiency, appropriateness, and cost benefit of the program.
- Recommend and implement modifications to better meet the needs of the community.
- Share findings and recommendations with community members and stakeholders.
- Ongoing evaluation is necessary in order to ensure program success (sustainability) and meet the changing needs of the community.

## STRATEGIES AND BARRIERS

### HELPFUL STRATEGIES
- Thorough assessment
- Accurate interpretation of data
- Collaboration with community partners
- Effective outreach and communication patterns
- Sufficient resources
- Logical planning
- Skilled leadership

### BARRIERS
- Inadequate assessment
- Inadequate or misconstrued data
- No involvement with community partners
- Impaired communication
- Inadequate resources
- Lack of planning
- Poor leadership

# Application Exercises

1. A nurse is preparing to conduct a windshield survey. Which of the following data should the nurse collect as a component of this assessment? (Select all that apply.)

   A. Ethnicity of community members
   B. Individuals who hold power within the community
   C. Natural community boundaries
   D. Prevalence of disease
   E. Presence of public protection

2. A nurse is completing a needs assessment and beginning analysis of data. Which of the following actions should the nurse take first?

   A. Determine health patterns within collected data.
   B. Compile collected data into a database.
   C. Ensure data collection is complete.
   D. Identify health needs of the local community.

3. A nurse is planning a community health program. Which of the following actions should the nurse include as part of the evaluation plan?

   A. Determine availability of resources to initiate the plan.
   B. Gain approval for the program from local leaders.
   C. Establish a timeline for implementation of interventions.
   D. Compare program impact to similar programs.

4. A nurse is conducting a community assessment. Which of the following data collection methods is the nurse using when having direct conversations with individual members of the community?

   A. Key informant interviews
   B. Participant observation
   C. Focus groups
   D. Health surveys

5. A nurse is collecting data to identify health needs in the local community. Which of the following examples should the nurse identify as secondary data? (Select all that apply.)

   A. Birth statistics
   B. Previous health survey results
   C. Windshield survey
   D. Community forum
   E. Health records

---

## PRACTICE Active Learning Scenario

A nurse collects the following data during a community assessment.

- Low crime rate
- Curbside garbage pick-up
- Increased incidence of low infant birth weight
- Small amount of litter along the road
- Public transportation that operates 24 hr/day, 7 days/week
- Older playground equipment in need of repair
- High prevalence of diabetes mellitus
- Recreational trails that are in need of maintenance

Use the ATI Active Learning Template: Basic Concept to complete this item.

**UNDERLYING PRINCIPLES:** Identify possible methods of collecting the data resulting from the nurse's community assessment.

**NURSING INTERVENTIONS**

- Name one action the nurse should take as part of the diagnosis phase of program development.
- Name three actions the nurse should take as part of the planning phase of program development.

# Application Exercises Key

1. A. **CORRECT:** The nurse should identify the ethnicity of the people visible in the community as a component of a windshield survey.

   B. Individuals who hold power are identified through formal and informal observations of community activities as a participant observer.

   C. **CORRECT:** The nurse should identify natural community boundaries as a component of a windshield survey.

   D. Prevalence of disease is incorrect. Disease prevalence is a component of secondary data and is identified through morbidity rates of the community.

   E. **CORRECT:** The nurse should identify the presence of public protection, such as police, fire, and animal control, as a component of a windshield survey.

   Ⓝ *NCLEX® Connection: Health Promotion and Maintenance, Health Promotion/Disease Prevention*

2. A. In order to determine health patterns within collected data, the nurse must take another action first.

   B. **CORRECT:** In order to adequately and appropriately analyze collected data, the nurse must first compile collected data into a database.

   C. In order to ensure data collection is complete, the nurse must take another action first.

   D. In order to identify health needs of the local community, the nurse must take another action first.

   Ⓝ *NCLEX® Connection: Management of Care, Establishing Priorities*

3. A. The nurse should determine availability of resources to initiate the program as part of the assessment phase. However, when evaluating sustainability of the program, the nurse should determine whether resources are available for continuing the program.

   B. The nurse should gain approval for the program from local leaders as part of the preplanning phase because plans for the program should not move forward without adequate community support.

   C. The nurse establishes a timeline for implementation of interventions after determining and selecting the best strategies for meeting the program's goals and objectives.

   D. **CORRECT:** The nurse should include a comparison of program impact to similar programs as part of the evaluation plan. This comparison assists with determining the efficiency of the program.

   Ⓝ *NCLEX® Connection: Health Promotion and Maintenance, Health Screening*

4. A. **CORRECT:** Informant interviews are direct conversations with individual community members for the purpose of obtaining ideas and opinions.

   B. Participant observation is observing formal or informal community activities and does not involve direct conversations with individual community members.

   C. Focus groups are directed talks with a representative sample of a community, and do not involve direct conversations with individual community members.

   D. Surveys are specific questions asked in a written format and do not involve direct conversations with individual community members.

   Ⓝ *NCLEX® Connection: Health Promotion and Maintenance, Health Promotion/Disease Prevention*

5. A. **CORRECT:** Birth statistics are an example of secondary data the nurse should review.

   B. **CORRECT:** Previous health survey results are an example of secondary data the nurse should review.

   C. Windshield surveys are a method of collecting direct data.

   D. Community forums are a method of collecting direct data.

   E. **CORRECT:** Health records are an example of secondary data the nurse should review.

   Ⓝ *NCLEX® Connection: Health Promotion and Maintenance, Health Promotion/Disease Prevention*

## PRACTICE Answer

*Using the ATI Active Learning Template: Basic Concept*

### UNDERLYING PRINCIPLES

- Curbside garbage pick-up: windshield survey, key informant interview, focus group
- Increased incidence of low infant birth weight: secondary data from health statistics
- Small amount of litter along the road: windshield survey
- Public transportation that operates 24 hr/day, 7 days/week: windshield survey, key informant interview
- Older playground equipment in need of repair: windshield survey, key informant interview, focus group
- High prevalence of diabetes mellitus: secondary data from health statistics
- Recreational trails that are in need of maintenance: windshield survey, key informant interview, focus group

### NURSING INTERVENTIONS

Diagnosis phase
- Analyze collected data to determine health needs within the local community.
- Work with community members, local health professionals and administrators to develop priorities and establish outcomes for identified health needs.

Planning phase
- Determine possible solutions to meet health needs of the community and select the best option.
- Establish goals and objectives for the selected solution.
- Select strategies/interventions to meet the objectives.
- Establish a timeline for implementation of interventions.
- Identify resources that are available, and resources that are needed, to implement strategies.
- Determine funding opportunities for needed interventions and develop a budget.
- Plan for program evaluation.

Ⓝ *NCLEX® Connection: Health Promotion and Maintenance, Health Promotion/Disease Prevention*

# ⓝ NCLEX® Connections

When reviewing the following chapter, keep in mind the relevant topics and tasks of the NCLEX outline, in particular:

## Client Needs: Safety and Infection Control

**ACCIDENT/ERROR/INJURY PREVENTION:** Identify deficits that may impede client safety.

**HOME SAFETY:** Educate client on home safety issues.

## Client Needs: Health Promotion and Maintenance

**DEVELOPMENTAL STAGES AND TRANSITIONS** Assist client to cope with life transitions.

Modify approaches to care in accordance with the client's developmental stage.

**HEALTH PROMOTION/DISEASE PREVENTION:** Assess and teach clients about health risks based on family, population, and/or community characteristics.

## Client Needs: Psychosocial Integrity

**END OF LIFE CARE:** Provide end of life care and education to clients.

**FAMILY DYNAMICS:** Evaluate resources available to assist family functioning.

**RELIGIOUS AND SPIRITUAL INFLUENCES ON HEALTH:** Assess psychosocial, spiritual, and occupational factors affecting care and plan interventions.

iron and calcium ↑absorption of lead.


Allergic to yeast = Ø Hep. B.

## CHAPTER 4 · *Practice Settings and Aggregates*

Community health nurses practice in diverse settings. They practice as home health nurses, hospice nurses, occupational health nurses, faith community nurses, school nurses, and forensic nurses.

Aggregates receive services from community health nurses. These include individuals from infancy to death, families, and groups within the community.

It is important to be aware of health disparities of each group (significant differences in health status) and to minimize those disparities when possible. Health disparities can be linked to gender, ethnicity, race, education, and income differences. Minority populations have a health disparity in relation to quality of care. Individuals who are of a minority tend to receive lower-quality health care regardless of the type of condition or other economic factors.

## *Practice settings*

### HOME HEALTH

Community health nurses provide health care services to clients where they reside. This includes traditional homes, assisted living facilities, and nursing homes.
- When making a visit to a client's home, the nurse should always take measures to ensure her own safety.
- The nurse is a guest in the client's home and should respect the values of the client and household members.
- Community health nursing care in the home setting is used to target specific at-risk individuals and groups.
- Community health nurses assist clients to transition from one level of care to another.
- Working as part of an interprofessional team is essential to providing holistic care. Qᵗᶜ
  - The interprofessional team provides care for the client in the home and is comprised of nurses, physical therapists, occupational therapists, home health aides, social workers, and dietitians.
  - The primary care provider prescribes services that are then usually coordinated by the home health nurse.

- The home health nurse functions as educator, provider of skilled nursing interventions, and coordinator of care. The nurse must consider the client assignment for each day and prioritize the order of visits.
  - Many clients leave the hospital in just a few days and are still very ill.
  - These clients and their family members need skilled services and education about the disease process, prescribed medications, and future implications of their illnesses.

SKILLED SERVICES INCLUDE:
- Skilled assessment
- Wound care
- Laboratory draws
- Medication education and administration
- Parenteral nutrition
- IV fluids and medication
- Central line care
- Urinary catheter insertion and maintenance
- Coordination, delegation and supervision of various other participants in health services

### *Omaha System model*

Nurses caring for individuals, families, and communities under home health and hospice care often use the Omaha System model to implement the nursing process. The framework is also used in many electronic health record systems.

STEPS OF THE OMAHA SYSTEM Qᴸ
- Collecting and assessing data
- Stating the problem
- Identifying an admission problem rating using a problem classification scheme
- Planning and intervening
- Re-rating problems during the span of care delivery and at discharge
- Evaluating the end problem outcome

## LIVING ENVIRONMENT

The home health nurse must evaluate the living environment for safety, paying close attention to nonsecure rugs, electrical outlets, and extension cords; the use of oxygen; low lighting; the need for safety devices in the bathroom; and other potential environmental hazards. Qˢ

Older adults are at a particular risk for falls. Ⓖ

QUESTIONS TO ASK
- Does the client have food in the house to eat?
- Is there help with household activities?
- Does the client live alone?
- Who is the client's support system?
- Is the client able to set up and dispense his own medication?
- Does the client have access to health care?

## CLIENT EDUCATION

Home health nurses provide follow-up care after an acute hospital stay. They must educate the client and the family regarding complications or adverse reactions.

- These instructions can include when to contact the agency, emergency room, or provider.
- Information and resources for families and clients can provide support in dealing with illness.

Providing education encourages clients to be independent and involved in their own care. It also allows families to be involved in the care and decision-making regarding their family members.

## HOSPICE

Hospice care focuses on enhancing the quality of life through the provision of palliative care, supporting the client and family through the dying process, and providing bereavement support to the family following the client's death.

- Clients can receive hospice care in a variety of settings, including the home, hospice centers, hospitals, and long-term care settings.
- Hospice care is a comprehensive care delivery system for clients who are terminally ill. Further medical care aimed toward a cure is stopped. The focus becomes relief of pain and suffering, as well as enhancing quality of life.
- The hospice nurse provides care for the client and the client's entire family. Hospice care includes skilled, direct services and indirect care coordination. **Q**pcc
- Hospice care uses an interprofessional approach.
- Controlling manifestations of the medical problem and dying process is a priority.
- The provider directs hospice care services which are then managed by the nurse.
- Volunteers are used for nonmedical care.
- Postmortem bereavement services are offered for the family.
- Helping the family transition from an expectation of recovery to acceptance of death is an important aspect of providing hospice care. The hospice nurse can continue to work with the family for up to 1 year following the death of the client.

## OCCUPATIONAL HEALTH

All work environments have associated risks. Health care in the workplace seeks to both promote health and prevent occupational illness and injury. Through improvement and maintenance of health, workplace expenditures are decreased by less sick time use, fewer workers' compensation claims, and decreased use of group health coverage.

- Nurses function in numerous roles within workplace settings and are challenged to provide cost-effective and high-quality care. In this effort it is essential for the occupational health nurse to develop partnerships with workplace administration, industrial hygienists, safety specialists, occupational medicine physicians, human resource departments, union representatives, and health insurance agencies. **Q**тс
- The occupational health nurse works to promote a healthy work environment to foster the health and safety of workers **Q**s
  - Assessing risks for work-related illness and injury
  - Planning and delivering health and safety services in the workplace
  - Collaborating with community health care providers
  - Facilitating health promotion activities that lead to a more productive workforce
- This autonomous specialty entails making independent nursing judgments when providing care to the workforce aggregate.

## SUSCEPTIBILITY

In assessing risk for work-related illness and injury, the nurse should keep in mind the following factors affecting susceptibility to illness and injury.

HOST FACTORS: Worker characteristics, such as job inexperience, age, and pregnancy

AGENT FACTORS
- Biological agents: viruses, bacteria, fungi, blood-borne, airborne pathogens
- Chemical agents: asbestos, smoke
- Mechanical agents: musculoskeletal or other strains from repetitive motions, poor workstation-worker fit, lifting heavy loads
- Physical agents: temperature extremes, vibrations, noise, radiation, lighting
- Psychological agents: threats to psychological or social well-being resulting in work-related stress, burnout, violence

ENVIRONMENTAL FACTORS
- Physical factors: heat, odor, ventilation, pollution
- Social factors: sanitation, overcrowding
- Psychological factors: addictions, stress

## RESPONSIBILITIES

Occupational health nurses' roles and responsibilities include the following.

**Primary prevention:** Teaching good nutrition and knowledge of health hazards, and providing information on immunizations, and use of protective equipment.

**Secondary prevention:** Identifying workplace hazards, early detection through health surveillance and screening, prompt treatment, counseling and referral, and prevention of further limitations.

**Tertiary prevention:** Restoration of health through rehabilitation strategies and limited-duty programs.

## EXPOSURE TO HAZARDS

An occupational health history provides the framework for a nurse to begin to assess a worker for possible exposure to health hazards.
- The goal is to identify agents and host factors that place the worker at risk, identify ways to eliminate or minimize exposure, and prevent potential health problems.
- Information elicited should include the following.
  - Current and past jobs
  - Current and past exposure to specific agents and any relationship of current manifestations to work activities
  - Any precipitating factors, such as underlying illness, previous injuries, and healthy or unhealthy habits

## SITE WALK-THROUGH

A work site walk-through or survey is also part of a workplace assessment. The occupational health nurse should focus on the following.
- Observation of work processes and materials
- Job requirements
- Actual and potential hazards
- Employee work practices: hygiene, waste disposal, housekeeping
- Incidence/prevalence of work-related illness/injuries
- Control strategies to eliminate exposures

## CONTROL STRATEGIES

Control strategies are designed to reduce future exposures based upon results from investigations into work-related illness/injury. Control strategies often include the following.
- Engineering
- Altering work practices
- Providing personal protective equipment and education to prevent future injuries
- Workplace monitoring
- Health screening
- Employee-assistance programs
- Job-task analysis
- Design, risk management, and emergency preparedness

## PROTECTION

### From violence
- Work can be frustrating and contribute to stress, resulting in aggression and violence against others.
- Be aware of jobs that are repetitive, boring, or physically and psychologically draining can help to identify workers who might feel tired, angry, and generally inadequate.
- Nurses can refer such workers to employee-assistance programs that provide confidential counseling and referrals to other professional services if needed.

### From work-related injuries

Related to falls, environmental hazards, and burns. Nurses can use research and trend analysis to improve working conditions by eliminating or minimizing hazards and potential problems. Q EBP

ADDITIONAL STRATEGIES
- Provide safety and health education programs to workers.
- Develop health policy focused on ensuring effective employee health and safety.
- Design strategies to prevent work-related accidents/injuries.
- Keeping abreast of Occupational Health and Safety Administration (OSHA) standards and resource programs.
- Working to influence legislation aimed at workers/workplace health protection.

## OCCUPATIONAL HEALTH AND LEGISLATION

### Occupational Safety and Health Act of 1970

**Occupational Health and Safety Administration (OSHA):** Develops and enforces workplace health regulations to protect the safety and health of workers. Provides education to employers about workplace health and safety.

**National Institute for Occupational Safety and Health (NIOSH):** A part of the Centers for Disease Control and prevention, it focuses on identification of workplace hazards and research for prevention of work-related injury and illness. Provides education to safety and health professionals about workplace safety.

**National Advisory Committee on Occupational Safety and Health (NACOSH):** The advisory committee is made up of 12 members representing labor, occupational health, and safety professions, and the general public. The committee's purpose is to advise the secretaries of labor and health and human services on policies and programs that affect occupational safety and health.

### Workers' compensation acts

State-level legislation that regulates financial compensation to workers suffering from injuries or illness resulting from the workplace.

workers' compensation is a state-run program.

# FAITH COMMUNITY

The faith community nurse works with individuals, families, and faith communities who share common faith traditions. Most religions have practices that are important to health and healing, and many follow specific practices when caring for an ill or dying member.

- Members of faith communities (congregants) represent the entire lifespan and all family types. This offers nurses the opportunity to work with a diverse population within the same setting.
- Faith community nurses provide interventions to individuals and groups in homes, congregational meeting places, acute or long-term care facilities or through schools.
- The practice of faith community nursing is governed by each state's nurse practice act and standards of practice.
- Nursing interventions are based on spiritual, physical, emotional, and social dimensions.
- Faith community nurses must be aware of faith and belief practices of the congregants served. Caring and spirituality are central among faith-based organizations.

## CIRCLE MODEL OF SPIRITUAL CARE Qᴘᴄᴄ

- **C:** Caring
- **I:** Intuition
- **R:** Respect for religious beliefs and practices
- **C:** Caution
- **L:** Listening
- **E:** Emotional support

## Missionary nurse

Missionary nursing seeks to promote health and prevent disease by meeting spiritual, physical, and emotional needs of people across the globe. These nurses can be career missionaries, or can serve as short-term, volunteer, or part-time missionaries.

Cultural and language barriers often affect the provision of care. Collaboration within the community is essential in meeting goals.

## Parish nurse

Parish nurses promote the health and wellness of populations of faith communities. The population often includes church members and individuals and groups in the geographical community.

Parish nurses work closely with pastoral care staff, professional health care members, and lay volunteers to provide a holistic approach to healing (body, mind, and spirit). Qᴛᴄ

## FUNCTIONS OF THE PARISH NURSE

- Personal health counseling (health-risk appraisals, spiritual assessments, support for numerous acute and chronic, actual and potential health problems)
- Health education (available resources, classes, individual and group teaching)
- Liaison between faith community and local resources
- Facilitating support groups
- Spiritual support (help identify spiritual strengths for coping)

# SCHOOL

School nursing encompasses many roles.

**Case manager:** Coordinates comprehensive services for children who have complex health needs.

**Community outreach:** Strives to meet the needs of all school-age children by cooperative planning and collaboration between the educational system and other community agencies.

**Consultant:** Assists students, families, and personnel in information gathering and decision-making about a variety of health needs and resources.

**Counselor:** Supports students on a wide variety of health needs. Can provide grief counseling.

**Direct caregiver:** Provides nursing care to ill or injured children at school.

**Health educator:** Helps prepare children, families, school personnel, and the community to make well-informed health decisions.

**Researcher:** Contributes to the base of knowledge for school health and educational needs. Qᴏɪ

## LEVELS OF PREVENTION

### Primary prevention

**Assess the knowledge base regarding health issues.**
Teach health promotion practices.
- Hand hygiene and tooth-brushing
- Healthy food choices
- Injury prevention, including seat belt use and bike, fire and water safety
- Substance use prevention
- Immunizations
- Disease prevention

**Assess the immunization status of all children.**
Maintain current records of required immunizations.

### Secondary prevention

**Assess children who become ill or injured at school.**
Provide care to children who have the following.
- Headaches
- Stomach pain, diarrhea
- Anxiety over being separated from parents
- Minor injuries (cuts or bruises) that occur at school

**Assess all children, faculty, and staff during emergencies.**
- Provide emergency care such as first aid, early defibrillation with AED and CPR.
- Create emergency plans for children who have a potential for anaphylactic reactions or other health problems that could result in an emergency situation.
- Maintain inventory of emergency supply equipment and secure medications.

**Perform screening for early detection of disease and initiate referrals as appropriate.**
- Vision and hearing
- Height and weight
- Oral health
- Scoliosis
- Infestations (lice)
- General physical examinations

**Assess children to detect child abuse or neglect.**
The school nurse is required by state law to officially report all suspected cases of child abuse/neglect.

**Assess children for evidence of mental illness, suicide, and violence.**
Identify children at risk.

**Respond to school crisis and disasters**
- Develop a crisis plan.
- Act as a first responder or triage the injured.
- Participate in drills.
- Counsel and debrief.

## Tertiary prevention

**Assess children who have disabilities.**
- Participate in developing the individual education plan (IEP) for children who have disabilities.
- Work with child/family to develop and achieve long-term outcomes.

**Assess children who have long-term health needs at school.**

**Provide nursing care for children who have chronic disorders, including asthma, diabetes mellitus, and cystic fibrosis.**
Administer medication per provider's prescription.
- The prescribed medication should be in the original bottle and stored in a secure place.
- Written consent by the parents for medication administration is required.
- Provide care to children who have specific health needs, including the following.
  - Urinary catheterizations
  - Dressing changes
  - IV line monitoring/medication administration
  - Tracheostomy suctioning
  - Tube feeding administration

**Provide ongoing care for adolescent parents or adolescents who are pregnant.**
- Assist in pregnancy identification
- Provide parenting education
- Educate adolescents on prevention of future pregnancies

## COMPONENTS OF COORDINATED SCHOOL HEALTH PROGRAMS

**Health education:** Inclusion of health concepts in courses of study for children in pre-K through grade 12

**Physical education:** Promoting physical activity in school

**Health services:** Providing health services in school by qualified professionals (nurses, physicians, dentists, allied health professionals)

**Nutrition services:** Providing access to meals that accommodate the health and nutrition needs of all children

**Counseling, psychological, and social services:** Providing services that improve the mental, emotional, and social health of students, as well as the overall school

**Promotion of a healthy and safe school environment:** Reducing tobacco use and violence in schools

**Health promotion for staff:** Promoting activities that encourage health promotion and disease prevention behaviors among the school's faculty and staff

**Facilitation of family/community involvement:** Promoting collaboration between the school, parents/caregivers, and community resources

## FORENSICS

Injury is a common cause of altered health that is preventable. Reducing the incidence of injury and promoting recovery reduces the financial burden of the condition. Qs

Forensic nurses care for perpetrators of injury as well as victims of sexual assault, substance use related injuries, human trafficking, physical abuse, gang violence, disaster, and accidental injuries.
- Forensic nursing combines nursing knowledge with knowledge of the criminal justice system, and epidemiological knowledge about findings of intentional injury.
- Forensic nurses work in a variety of settings, including clinics, emergency departments, law enforcement agencies, mental health facilities, and correctional facilities.
- Safety is the primary principle of forensic nursing care. Other key principles include respect, beneficence, nonmaleficence, caring, justice, truth, and the use of intuition.
- Many forensic nursing roles require advanced education and certification. Credentialing in forensic nursing is available for the sexual assault nurse examiner (SANE) and advanced practice forensic nurses.
- The SANE collects detailed medical, physical, and emotional data from clients following a sexual assault, manages samples, and provides support to clients. A SANE often testifies in legal proceedings related to findings of client assessment.

## LEVELS OF PREVENTION

**Primary prevention:** Develop and implement injury prevention programs (sudden infant death syndrome [SIDS], sexual assault).

**Secondary prevention**
- Examine victims of crime for indicators of intentional injury.
- Provide direct care to both the client following a sexual assault and perpetrator
- Collect and preserve evidence from possible crimes, using written and picture documentation.

**Tertiary prevention**
- Provide treatment to incarcerated individuals.
- Liaison between clients following trauma, medical care facilities, and the legal community to minimize the burden of trauma on the client.
- Connect clients with community resources after injury (mental health counseling, physical rehabilitation).

# Aggregates of the community

## CHILDREN (BIRTH TO 12 YEARS) AND ADOLESCENTS

## HEALTH CONCERNS/ LEADING CAUSES OF DEATH

### CHILDREN
- Perinatal conditions/congenital anomalies
- SIDS
- Motor vehicle/other unintentional injuries

### ADOLESCENTS
- Motor vehicle/other unintentional injuries
- Homicide
- Suicide

## SCREENING/PREVENTIVE SERVICES

### CHILDREN
- Height/weight
- Vision and hearing
- At birth: hemoglobinopathy, phenylalanine level, T4, and TSH
- Immunization status: check the Centers for Disease Control and Prevention (CDC) , www.cdc.gov, for current administration schedules
- Lead exposure
- Cholesterol and triglyceride levels
- Dental health

### ADOLESCENTS
- Height/weight
- Dental health
- Rubella serology/immunization history (females)
- Substance use disorders, including tobacco
- Immunization status (www.cdc.gov)
- Mental health screenings
- Cholesterol and triglyceride levels
- Vision and hearing

## NATIONAL HEALTH GOALS Q℮ᴮᴾ

### CHILDREN
- REDUCTIONS IN
  - Dental caries
  - Obesity
  - Exposure to secondhand smoke
- INCREASES IN
  - Newborn blood spot screenings and follow-up testing
  - Access to a medical home
  - Schools that require health education
  - Childhood immunizations
  - Use of child safety restraints
  - Physical activity

### ADOLESCENTS
- REDUCTIONS IN
  - Violent crimes
  - Initiation of tobacco use
  - Obesity
  - Deaths related to motor vehicle crashes
- INCREASES IN
  - Schools with a breakfast program
  - Participation in extracurricular activities
  - Wellness checkups within prior 12 months
  - Physical activity

## COMMUNITY EDUCATION

### CHILDREN
- Anticipatory guidance
- Breastfeeding
- Sleeping positions
- Nutrition
- Physical activity
- Substance use disorders
- Dental hygiene/health
- Skin protection
- Injury prevention including car, fire, and water safety; helmet use; poison control; and CPR training

### ADOLESCENTS
- Anticipatory guidance
- Substance use disorders
- Sexual behavior
- Nutrition, especially calcium intake for female clients
- Physical activity
- Skin protection
- Injury prevention including car, fire, and firearm safety

<table>
<tr><th>WOMEN</th><th>MEN</th></tr>
</table>

## HEALTH CONCERNS/ LEADING CAUSES OF DEATH

- Reproductive health
  - Childbearing
  - Menopause
  - Osteoporosis
- Heart disease
- Diabetes mellitus
- Malignant neoplasm (breast, cervical, ovarian, colorectal)

## SCREENING/PREVENTIVE SERVICES

- Height/weight
- Blood pressure
- Cholesterol (ages 45 to 65)
- Dental health
- Pap smear test
- Mammogram/clinical breast exam
- Fecal occult blood test/sigmoidoscopy (50 years and older)
- Rubella serology/vaccination history (childbearing years)
- Immunization status: check the CDC, www.cdc.gov, for current administration schedules
- Diabetes mellitus
- HIV
- Skin cancer

## NATIONAL HEALTH GOALS Q<sub>EBP</sub>

### REDUCTIONS IN

- Diseases involving bone, such as osteoporosis
- Death from cancer such as breast, ovarian, and cervical
- Sexual violence

### INCREASES IN

- Number of planned pregnancies versus unplanned
- Those who receive early and adequate prenatal care
- The number of mothers who breastfeed
- Ability to identify warning indicators of a heart attack and stroke
- Abstinence from alcohol, nicotine and other substances among pregnant women

## COMMUNITY EDUCATION

- Nutrition
- STI prevention
- Substance use disorders
- Breast self-examination
- Skin protection
- HIV prevention
- Injury prevention including car, fire safety, and violence

## HEALTH CONCERNS/ LEADING CAUSES OF DEATH

- Heart disease
- Malignant neoplasm (prostate, testicular, skin, colorectal)
- Unintentional injuries
- Lung disease
- Liver disease

## SCREENING/PREVENTIVE SERVICES

- Height/weight
- Blood pressure
- Dental health
- Digital rectal exam
- Fecal occult blood test/sigmoidoscopy (50 years and older)
- Immunization status: check the CDC, www.cdc.gov, for current administration schedules
- Diabetes mellitus
- HIV
- Skin cancer
- Cholesterol (ages 45 to 65 years)

## NATIONAL HEALTH GOALS Q<sub>EBP</sub>

### REDUCTIONS IN

- Death from cancer specific to men, such as prostate
- Incidence of HIV and AIDS
- Fatal and nonfatal injuries

### INCREASES IN

- Participation in aerobic and muscle-strengthening activities
- Ability to identify warning indicators of a heart attack and stroke

## COMMUNITY EDUCATION

- Nutrition
- Self-testicular exam
- Skin protection
- Substance use disorders
- HIV prevention
- Injury prevention including car, fire and firearm safety, and violence

## OLDER ADULTS ©

### HEALTH CONCERNS/ LEADING CAUSES OF DEATH

- Heart disease
- Malignant neoplasm
- Cerebrovascular disease
- Chronic obstructive pulmonary disease
- Pneumonia and influenza
- Substance use disorders

### SCREENING/PREVENTIVE SERVICES

- Blood pressure
- Height/weight
- Dental health
- Fecal occult blood test/sigmoidoscopy
- Mammogram/clinical breast exam (women)
- Pap smear test (women)
- Vision
- Hearing
- Substance use
- Immunization status (pneumococcal, influenza): check the CDC, www.cdc.gov, for current administration schedules
- Functional assessment (self-care abilities)
- Medication history
- Osteoporosis
- Diabetes mellitus
- Skin cancer

### NATIONAL HEALTH GOALS Q$_{EBP}$

REDUCTIONS IN
- Adults who have musculoskeletal concerns
- Older adults who have mental health concerns
- Hospitalizations due to heart failure
- Substance use in the older adult
- Sensory concerns such as hearing loss and cataracts
- Hip fractures among older adults
- Fall-related deaths

INCREASES IN
- Screenings for colorectal cancer
- Participation in organized health promotion activities
- Public reporting of elder abuse or neglect
- Older adults who maintain an active lifestyle
- Self-management of chronic health disorders

### COMMUNITY EDUCATION

- Substance use disorders
- Nutrition
- Exercise
- Dental health
- Sexual behavior
- Injury prevention
  - Car and fire safety
  - Fall prevention
  - Violence

## FAMILIES

The family as client is basic to community-oriented nursing practice. Community health nurses have a significant role to play in promoting healthy families.

A family consists of individuals who identify themselves as family members and have an interdependent relationship that provides emotional, financial, and/ or physical support. There are numerous structures and forms families can choose to take.
- Community health nurses must engage in community assessment, planning, development, and evaluation activities that are focused on family issues.
- Home visits provide community health nurses with the opportunity to observe the home environment and to identify barriers and supports to health-risk reduction. Q$_{PCC}$

### APPROACHES

The nurse can take several different approaches to nursing care of a family.

**Family as a component of society**
- Monitors how families interact with other institutions in a community (schools, medical facilities, congregations)
- Used to study and implement population-focused interventions (e.g. immunization campaigns for a disadvantaged population)

**Family as a system**
- Studies how interactions among family members affect the whole family function
- Used to promote family health by directing interventions toward the way family members interact with each other

**Family as client**
- Examines the family unit functioning first, then individual needs next
- Used to see how the family health is impacted by each individual's reaction to a health event

**Family as context**
- Focuses on an individual first, and the family next
- Used to promote the health and recovery of an individual, using the family as a resource for service and support

### CRISIS AND TRANSITIONS

Family crisis occurs when a family is not able to cope with an event. The family's resources are inadequate for the demands of the situation.

Transitions are times of risk for families.
- Transitions include birth or adoption of a child, death of a family member, child moving out of the home, marriage of a child, major illness, divorce, and loss of the main family income.
- These transitions require families to change behaviors, make new decisions, reallocate family roles, learn new skills, and learn to use new resources.

## CHARACTERISTICS OF HEALTHY FAMILIES

- Members communicate well and listen to each other.
- There is affirmation and support for all members.
- Members teach respect for others.
- There is a sense of trust.
- Members play and share humor together.
- Members interact with one another.
- Members participate in leisure activities together.
- Members share a religious foundation.
- Privacy of individuals is respected.
- There is a shared sense of responsibility.
- There are traditions and rituals.
- Members seek help for their problems.

## FAMILY HEALTH RISK APPRAISAL

### BIOLOGICAL HEALTH RISK ASSESSMENT

- Genograms are used to gather basic information about the family, relationships within the family, and health and illness patterns. Genomics involves the study of genetic information and how it is influenced and expressed. Providers can use genomic information to identify specific individual risks and provide appropriate prevention.
- Repetitions of diseases with a genetic component (cancer, heart disease, diabetes mellitus) can be identified.

ENVIRONMENTAL RISK: Ecomaps are used to identify family interactions with other groups and organizations. Information about the family's support network and social risk is gathered.

BEHAVIORAL RISK: Information is gathered about the family's health behavior, including health values, health habits, and health risk perceptions.

## NATIONAL HEALTH GOALS Q<sub>EBP</sub>

### REDUCTIONS IN

- Barriers to access
- Allergens within the home
- Families that are unable to have a child or maintain a pregnancy
- Passive smoke exposure
- Household hunger
- Intimate partner violence

### INCREASES IN

- Positive parenting
- Health education provided by an agency (Head Start, school system, college, places of employment, health departments)
- Home testing for radon
- Health insurance coverage
- Individuals who have a usual primary care provider

# Application Exercises

1. A nurse is talking to a client who asks for additional information about hospice. Which of the following statements should the nurse make?

   A. "Clients who require skilled nursing care at home qualify for hospice care."

   B. "One function of hospice is to provide teaching to clients about life-sustaining measures."

   C. "Hospice assists clients to develop the skills needed to care for themselves independently."

   D. "A component of hospice care is to control the client's manifestations."

2. A school nurse is scheduling visits with a physical therapist for a child who has cerebral palsy. In which of the following roles is the nurse functioning?

   A. Direct caregiver

   B. Consultant

   C. Case manager

   D. Counselor

3. An occupational health nurse is consulting with senior management of a local industrial facility. When discussing work-related illness and injury, the nurse should include which of the following factors as physical agents? (Select all that apply.)

   A. Noise

   B. Age

   C. Lighting

   D. Viruses

   E. Stress

4. A newly hired occupational health nurse at an industrial facility is performing an initial workplace assessment. Which of the following information should the nurse determine when conducting a work site survey?

   A. Work practices of employees

   B. Past exposure to specific agents

   C. Past jobs of individual employees

   D. Length of time working in current role

5. A school nurse is planning health promotion and disease prevention activities for the upcoming school year. In which of the following situations is the nurse planning a secondary prevention strategy?

   A. Placing posters with images of appropriate hand hygiene near restrooms

   B. Routinely checking students for pediculosis throughout the school year

   C. Implementing age-appropriate injury prevention programs for each grade level

   D. Working with a dietitian to determine carbohydrate counts for students who have diabetes mellitus

---

## PRACTICE Active Learning Scenario

A nurse is developing programs to promote the health of families in the local community. Use the ATI Active Learning Template: Basic Concept to complete this item.

RELATED CONTENT: Describe three characteristics of healthy families.

UNDERLYING PRINCIPLES
- Include two times families experience transition.
- Include two national health goals that apply to families.

NURSING INTERVENTIONS: Explain two strategies to improve the health of families.

# Application Exercises Key

1. A. Clients who require skilled nursing care at home qualify for home health.

   B. Home health can provide teaching to clients about life-sustaining measures. In hospice, medical care aimed toward a cure is stopped.

   C. Home health assists clients to develop the skills needed to care for themselves independently.

   D. **CORRECT:** Controlling the client's manifestations of medical problems or the dying process and improving quality of life are components of hospice care.

   (N) *NCLEX® Connection: Basic Care and Comfort, Non–Pharmacological Comfort Interventions*

2. A. In the role of direct caregiver, a school nurse provides illness and injury care to children at school.

   B. In the role of consultant, a school nurse provides information to families, administrators, teachers, and parent-teacher groups to encourage decisions that promote the health of the students.

   C. **CORRECT:** In the role of case manager, a school nurse coordinates comprehensive services for students who have complex health needs.

   D. In the role of counselor, a school nurse develops a trusting relationship with students and provides support on issues affecting their lives.

   (N) *NCLEX® Connection: Management of Care, Case Management*

3. A. **CORRECT:** The nurse manager should include noise as a physical agent when discussing work-related illness and injury.

   B. The nurse manager should include age as a host factor when discussing work-related illness and injury.

   C. **CORRECT:** The nurse manager should include lighting as a physical agent when discussing work-related illness and injury.

   D. The nurse manager should include viruses as a biological agent when discussing work-related illness and injury.

   E. The nurse manager should include stress as an outcome of psychological agents when discussing work-related illness and injury.

   (N) *NCLEX® Connection: Psychosocial Integrity, Stress Management*

4. A. **CORRECT:** The nurse should determine the work practices of employees when conducting a work site survey.

   B. The nurse should determine past exposure to specific agents when conducting an occupational health history on individual workers, not a work site survey.

   C. The nurse should determine past jobs of individual employees when conducting an occupational health history on individual workers, not a work site survey.

   D. The nurse should determine the length of time working in current role when conducting an occupational health history on individual workers, not a work site survey.

   (N) *NCLEX® Connection: Health Promotion and Maintenance, Health Promotion/Disease Prevention*

5. A. The nurse should place posters with images of appropriate hand hygiene near restrooms as a primary prevention strategy.

   B. **CORRECT:** Routinely checking students for pediculosis throughout the school year is a secondary prevention strategy the nurse can take.

   C. The nurse should implement age-appropriate injury-prevention programs for each grade level as a primary prevention activity.

   D. The nurse should work with the dietitian to determine carbohydrate counts for students who have diabetes mellitus as a tertiary prevention activity.

   (N) *NCLEX® Connection: Health Promotion and Maintenance, Health Screening*

---

## PRACTICE Answer

*Using the ATI Active Learning Template: Basic Concept*

### RELATED CONTENT
- Members communicate well and listen to each other.
- There is affirmation and support for all members.
- Members teach respect for others.
- There is a sense of trust.
- Members play and share humor together.
- Members interact with one another.
- Members participate in leisure activities together.
- Members share a religious foundation.
- Privacy of individuals is respected.
- There is a shared sense of responsibility.
- There are traditions and rituals.
- Members seek help for their problems.

### UNDERLYING PRINCIPLES
Times of transition
- Birth of a child
- Adoption of a child
- Death of a family member
- Child moving from the home
- Child getting married
- Major illness of a family member
- Divorce of a family member
- Loss of the main source of family income

National health goals
- Reductions in
  - Barriers to access
  - Allergens within the home
  - Families that are unable to have a child or maintain a pregnancy
  - Passive smoke exposure
  - Household hunger
  - Intimate partner violence
- Increases in
  - Positive parenting
  - Health education provided by an agency
  - Home testing for radon
  - Health insurance coverage
  - Individuals with a usual primary care provider

### NURSING INTERVENTIONS
- Identify barriers and supports to health-risk reduction.
- Assess safety during home visits.
- Identify and coordinate needed community resource referrals.
- Perform biological health risk assessments.
- Assess for environmental and behavioral risks.

(N) *NCLEX® Connection: Psychosocial Integrity, Family Dynamics*

When reviewing the following chapter, keep in mind the relevant topics and tasks of the NCLEX outline, in particular:

## Client Needs: Management of Care

**CASE MANAGEMENT:** Assess the client's need for materials and equipment.

**LEGAL RIGHTS AND RESPONSIBILITIES:** Identify legal issues affecting the client.

## Client Needs: Psychosocial Integrity

**ABUSE/NEGLECT:** Plan interventions for victims/suspected victims of abuse.

**CHEMICAL AND OTHER DEPENDENCIES/SUBSTANCE USE DISORDER:** Provide information on substance abuse diagnosis and treatment plan to the client.

**COPING MECHANISMS:** Assess the client's support systems and available resources.

## Client Needs: Basic Care and Comfort

**NON-PHARMACOLOGICAL COMFORT INTERVENTIONS:** Incorporate alternative/complementary therapies into client plan of care.

**NUTRITION AND ORAL HYDRATION:** Provide/maintain special diets based on the client diagnosis/ nutritional needs and cultural considerations.

# Care of Specific Populations

Community health nurses identify vulnerable populations and implement measures to improve health through direct care, improving access, and changing the physical environment, health care culture, and health policies.

Community health nurses can link vulnerable clients to relevant agencies and resources within a community (food banks, shelters, mental health centers) to meet client needs. Clients can require assistance with referrals or transportation.

Community health nurses care for many individuals who are members of specific populations and more prone to impaired health or negative outcomes associated with illness and disease.

## VULNERABLE POPULATIONS

These include individuals who are subject to issues such as the following.
- Violence
- Substance use disorders
- Mental health issues/illnesses
- Poverty and homelessness
- Rural residency
- Migrant employment
- Veteran status
- Disability

### OTHER FACTORS THAT CAN THREATEN HEALTH
- Low income
- Difficulty accessing health care
- Poor self-esteem
- Young or advanced age
- Chronic stress
- Environmental factors

## NATIONAL HEALTH GOALS

Goals to address for vulnerable populations include the following.
- Increasing the number of people who have a routine primary care provider
- Increasing the number of people who have health insurance
- Reducing the number of people who are unable to access or have a delay in accessing health care services and prescribed medications
- Reducing the number of people who have disabilities who report physical barriers to accessing health and wellness programs in the community

# Violence

## TYPES WITHIN COMMUNITIES

### Homicide

- Homicide is often related to substance use.
- Most homicides are committed by someone known to the victim and occur during an argument.
- Abuse often precedes homicide within families.
- Rates of homicide are increasing among adolescents more than in other age groups.

### Assault

- Males are more likely than females to be assaulted.
- Youths are at a significantly increased risk.

### Rape

- Rape is often unreported.
- Most incidences of rape are spousal (marital) or acquaintance (date) rape.
- Females are more likely than males to be raped. The risk of rape is increased in cities, between 8 p.m. and 2 a.m., on the weekends, and in the summer months.

### Suicide

- According to the CDC:
  - Rates of suicide are highest among individuals 45 to 64 years of age.
  - Females are more likely to attempt suicide; however, males are more likely to complete suicide.
  - Caucasians are more likely than other ethnic groups to commit suicide.
- Risk factors for suicide include depression or other mental health disorders, substance use, having access to a firearm, and intimate partner issues.

## Abuse

**PHYSICAL VIOLENCE** occurs when pain or harm results.
- **Toward an infant or child**, as is the case with shaken baby syndrome (caused by violent shaking of young infants)
- **Toward an intimate partner**, such as striking or strangling the partner
- **Toward an older adult** in the home (elder abuse), such as pushing an older adult parent and causing her to fall ⊙

**SEXUAL VIOLENCE** occurs when sexual contact takes place without consent.

**EMOTIONAL VIOLENCE**, which includes behavior that minimizes an individual's feelings of self-worth or humiliates, threatens, or intimidates a family member.

**NEGLECT** includes the failure to provide the following.
- **Physical care**, such as food, shelter, and hygiene
- **Emotional care** and/or stimulation necessary to achieve developmental milestones, such as speaking and interacting with a child
- **Education** for a child
- Needed **health or dental care**

### Economic maltreatment

- Failure to provide for the needs of a vulnerable person when adequate funds are available
- Unpaid bills when another person is managing the finances
- Theft of or misuse of money or property

## INDIVIDUAL ASSESSMENT FOR VIOLENCE

### INDIVIDUAL RISK FACTORS FOR VIOLENCE
- History of being abused or exposure to violence
- Low self-esteem
- Fear and distrust of others
- Poor self-control
- Inadequate social skills
- Minimal social support/isolation
- Immature motivation for marriage or childbearing
- Weak coping skills

### RECOGNIZING POTENTIAL CHILD ABUSE/NEGLECT
- Unexplained injury
- Unusual fear of the nurse and others
- Injuries/wounds not mentioned in history
- Fractures, including older healed fractures
- Presence of injuries/wounds/fractures in various stages of healing
- Subdural hematomas
- Trauma to genitalia
- Malnourishment or dehydration
- General poor hygiene or inappropriate dress for weather conditions
- Parent considers child to be a "bad child"

### RECOGNIZING POTENTIAL OLDER ADULT ABUSE ⊙
- Unexplained or repeated physical injuries
- Physical neglect and unmet basic needs
- Rejection of assistance by caregiver
- Financial mismanagement
- Withdrawal and passivity
- Depression

## COMMUNITY ASSESSMENT

### SOCIAL AND COMMUNITY VIOLENCE RISK FACTORS
- Work stress
- Unemployment
- Media exposure to violence
- Crowded living conditions
- Poverty
- Feelings of powerlessness
- Social isolation
- Lack of community resources (playgrounds, parks, theaters)

## STRATEGIES TO REDUCE SOCIETAL VIOLENCE Qs

### PRIMARY PREVENTION
- Teach alternative methods of conflict resolution, anger management, and coping strategies in community settings.
- Organize parenting classes to provide anticipatory guidance of expected age-appropriate behaviors, appropriate parental responses, and forms of discipline.
- Educate clients about community services that are available to provide protection from violence.
- Promote public understanding about the aging process and about safeguards to ensure a safe and secure environment for older adults in the community. ⊙
- Assist in removing or reducing factors that contribute to stress by referring caretakers of older adult clients to respite services, assisting an unemployed parent in finding employment, or increasing social support networks for socially isolated families.
- Encourage older adults and their families to safeguard their funds and property by getting more information about a financial representative trust, durable power of attorney, a representative payee, and joint tenancy.
- Teach individuals that no one has a right to touch or hurt another person, and make sure they know how to report cases of abuse.

### SECONDARY PREVENTION

- Identify and screen those at risk for abuse and individuals who are potential abusers.
- Assess and evaluate any unexplained bruises or injuries of any individual.
- Screen all pregnant women for potential abuse. This might be the one time in some women's lives that they can access the health care system on a regular basis.
- Refer sexual assault or rape survivors to a local emergency department for assessment by a sexual assault abuse team. Caution the client not to bathe following the assault because it will destroy physical evidence.
- Assess and counsel anyone contemplating suicide or homicide, and refer the individual to the appropriate services.
- Support and educate the offender, even though a report must be made.
- Assess and help offenders address and deal with the stressors that can be causing or contributing to the abuse, such as mental illness or substance use.
- Alert all involved about available resources within the community.
- Advocate for legislation designed to assist older adult independence and caregivers and to increase funding for programs that supply services to low-income, at-risk individuals.

### TERTIARY PREVENTION

- Establish parameters for long-term follow-up and supervision.
- Make resources in the community available to survivors of violence (telephone numbers of crisis lines and shelters).
- If court systems are involved, work with parents while the child is out of the home (in foster care).
- Refer to mental health professionals for long-term assistance.
- Provide grief counseling to families following the death of a family member to suicide or homicide.
- Develop support groups for caregivers and survivors of violence.

## CARING FOR CLIENTS WHO EXPERIENCE VIOLENCE QPCC

- Build trust and confidence with a client.
- Focus on the client rather than the situation.
- Assess for immediate danger.
- Provide emergency care as needed.
- Work with the client to develop a plan for safety.
- Make needed referrals for community services and legal options.
- If abuse has occurred, complete mandatory reporting, following state and agency guidelines.

## Substance use disorders

- Substance use disorders involve the maladaptive use of substances resulting in threats to an individual's health or social and economic functioning.
- Substance use disorders have significant effects on family dynamics, and often lead to codependency.
- Substance use disorders negatively affect family life, public safety, and the economy.
- Recovery from substance use disorders occurs over years and usually involves relapses. A strong support system, including 12-step programs and self-help groups for family members, is important.
- Community health nurses are front-line health professionals who are able to assist those who have substance use disorders.

## DEPENDENCE

Dependence is a pattern of pathological, compulsive use of substances and involves physiological and psychological dependence.

- Cardinal indicators of dependence include manifestations of tolerance and withdrawal.
- Denial is also a primary indication of dependence and can include the following.
  - Defensiveness
  - Lying about use
  - Minimizing use
  - Blaming or rationalizing use
  - Intellectualizing
  - "Going with the flow" (agreeing there is a problem, vowing to make a change, but the change doesn't occur)

## HEALTH PROBLEMS

Alcohol, tobacco, and other substance use disorders can cause multiple health problems, including the following.
- Low birth weight
- Congenital abnormalities
- Accidents
- Homicides
- Suicides
- Chronic diseases
- Violence

## ALCOHOL USE

- Alcohol is the most commonly used substance in the U.S. It is socially acceptable, as well as easily accessible.
- Alcohol is a depressant. Alcohol dulls the senses to outside stimulation and sedates the inhibitory centers in the brain.
- People who frequently and consistently drink alcohol develop a tolerance, an increased requirement for alcohol to achieve the desired effect.

## EFFECT OF ALCOHOL

- The direct effect of alcohol is determined by the blood alcohol level.
- The body processes alcohol dependent on several factors.
  - Size and weight of the drinker
  - Gender (affects metabolism)
  - Carbonation (increases absorption)
  - Time elapsed during alcohol consumption
  - Food in the stomach
  - The drinker's emotional state
  - Type of alcohol
- Excess alcohol that is not metabolized circulates in the blood and affects the central nervous system and the brain.

## WITHDRAWAL

- Following prolonged use, manifestations of alcohol withdrawal appears within 4 to 12 hr.
- It is important to determine the time of the last drink the client ingested in order to accurately monitor for manifestations of withdrawal.

### MANIFESTATIONS OF WITHDRAWAL

- Irritability
- Tremors
- Nausea
- Vomiting
- Headaches
- Diaphoresis
- Anxiety
- Sleep disturbances
- Tachycardia
- Elevated blood pressure

## TOBACCO USE

- Smoking is the most important preventable cause of death in the U.S., according to the Centers for Disease Control and Prevention. Q EBP
- Nicotine is a stimulant that temporarily creates a feeling of alertness and energy. Repeated use to avoid the subsequent "down" that will follow this period of stimulation leads to a vicious cycle of use.
- Tolerance to nicotine develops quickly.
- Cigarette smoking results in deep inhalation of smoke, which poses the greatest health risk (cancer, cardiovascular disease, respiratory disease).
  - Cigars, pipes, and smokeless tobacco increase the risk of cancers of the lips, mouth, and throat.
  - Passive smoking (exposure to secondhand smoke) poses considerable health risks (respiratory disease, lung cancer) to nonsmokers.

## OTHER SUBSTANCES

**Marijuana** has a low level of toxicity. Although it is legal in some states, it is considered the most commonly used illegal substance in the U.S. Users can develop tolerance and dependence with long-term use, but withdrawal manifestations are minimal.

**Other stimulants** include caffeine, amphetamines, methamphetamines, and cocaine.

**Other depressants** include barbiturates, benzodiazepines, chloral hydrate, and GHB.

**Opiates** include morphine, heroin, codeine, and fentanyl.

**Hallucinogens (psychedelics)** produce anxiety, paranoia, impaired judgment, and hallucinations. Some examples are lysergic acid diethylamide (LSD), phencyclidine (PCP), and MDMA (ecstasy).

**Inhalants** are volatile substances that are inhaled (huffed). Death can result from acute cardiac dysrhythmias or asphyxiation.

## INDIVIDUAL ASSESSMENT Q PCC

- Establish rapport with the client. Pose questions in a matter-of-fact tone. Be nonjudgmental. Communicate that the purpose of questioning is because of the effects that different practices can have on an individual's health. Use therapeutic communication.
- Seek information about specific substances used, methods of use, and the quantity (packs, ounces) and frequency of use.
- Elicit information about consequences experienced (blackouts, overdoses, injuries to self/others, legal or social difficulties).
- Determine if the individual perceives a substance use problem.
- Discuss the individual's history of previous rehabilitation experiences.
- Gather family history of substance use and social exposure to other substance users.

## PHYSICAL ASSESSMENT FINDINGS

**VITAL SIGNS:** Varies depending on substance being used.

**APPEARANCE:** Individual can appear disheveled with an unsteady gait.

**EYES:** Pupils can appear dilated or pinpoint, red, and with poor eye contact.

**SKIN:** Can be diaphoretic, cool, and/or clammy. Needle track marks or spider angiomas can be visible.

**NOSE:** Can be runny, congested, red, and/or cauliflower-shaped.

**TREMORS:** Fine or coarse tremors can be present.

## STRATEGIES TO REDUCE SUBSTANCE USE DISORDERS

### PRIMARY PREVENTION

- Increase public awareness, particularly among young people, regarding the hazards and risks of dependence associated with substance use (e.g., public education campaigns, school education programs).
- Encourage development of life skills.
- Assist in the formation of parental action and awareness groups, such as Mothers Against Drunk Driving (MADD).

### SECONDARY PREVENTION

- Identify at-risk individuals and assist them to reduce sources of stress, including possible referral to social services to eliminate financial difficulties or other sources of stress.
- Screen individuals for substance use disorders.

### TERTIARY PREVENTION

- Assist the client to develop a plan to avoid high-risk situations and to enhance coping and lifestyle changes.
- Refer the client to community groups, such as Alcoholics Anonymous (AA) and Narcotics Anonymous (NA).
- Monitor pharmacological management (nicotine replacement therapy, methadone programs).
- Provide emotional support to recovering substance users and their families, including positive reinforcement.

## Mental health

National Alliance for the Mentally Ill (NAMI) is an advocacy group that works to reduce stigma and provide services for clients who have mental health disorders and their families.

## CHARACTERISTICS OF MENTAL HEALTH DISORDERS

- Occurs across the lifespan
- High risk of substance use disorders
- High suicide risk

## SPECIFIC DISORDERS

- Affective disorders (bipolar disorder, major depressive disorder)
- Anxiety disorders (obsessive-compulsive, panic, phobias, posttraumatic stress)
- Schizophrenia
- Dementia
- Conduct disorders
- Personality disorders

## FACTORS AFFECTING MENTAL HEALTH

- Individual coping abilities
- Stressful life events (exposure to violence, disasters)
- Social events (recent divorce, separation, unemployment, bereavement)
- Chronic health problems
- Stigma associated with seeking mental health services

## STRATEGIES FOR IMPROVING MENTAL HEALTH

### PRIMARY PREVENTION

- Provide education to populations regarding mental health issues.
- Teach stress-reduction techniques.
- Implement parenting classes.
- Organize bereavement support groups.
- Promote protective factors (coping abilities) and risk factor reduction.

### SECONDARY PREVENTION

- Screen to detect mental health disorders.
- Work directly with at-risk individuals, families, and groups through formation of a therapeutic relationship.
- Conduct crisis intervention.

### TERTIARY PREVENTION

- Perform medication monitoring.
- Provide mental health interventions.
- Make referrals to various groups of professionals, including support groups.
- Maintain the client's level of function to prevent relapse or frequent rehospitalization.
- Identify behavioral, environmental, and biological triggers that can lead to relapse.
- Assist the client in planning a regular lifestyle and minimizing sources of stress.
- Educate the client and family regarding medication adverse effects and potential interactions.

## Poverty and homelessness

- The federal poverty level is used to help determine which individuals can receive financial assistance (Medicaid, welfare).
- Individuals living in poverty are unable to pay for food, transportation, shelter, clothes, and medical care.
- Community regions that are characterized by poor housing, low employment rates, and increased rates of death and disease can be described as neighborhood poverty.
- Extreme poverty leads to inadequate housing and homelessness.
- Homeless individuals are those who do not have a regular nighttime residence, and can include individuals who temporarily reside in a shelter, institution, or on the street.
- Incidence and prevalence counts can be used to number homeless individuals. The number is often inaccurate due to difficultly locating homeless individuals who can be transient, staying with friends, or residing in difficult-to-access locations.

## POVERTY

### CHARACTERISTICS OF INDIVIDUALS EXPERIENCING POVERTY

- Insufficient insurance coverage
- High-risk work and living environments
- Poor nutrition
- Increased stress
- Less likely to engage in preventive activities or seek treatment for health problems
- Increased rate of chronic illness and accompanying physical limitations
- Increased morbidity and mortality rates

## HOMELESSNESS

### HOMELESS POPULATION CHARACTERISTICS

- Adults who are unemployed, earn low wages, or are migrant workers
- Female heads of households
- Families with children (fastest-growing segment)
- People who have a mental illness (large segment)
- Veterans
- People who have substance use disorders
- Unaccompanied youth
- Adolescent runaways (high incidence of lesbian, gay, bisexual, and transgender [LGBT] adolescents)
- Intimate partner abuse survivors
- People who have HIV or AIDS
- Older adults who have no place to go and no support system ⓒ

### HEALTH ISSUES OF HOMELESS POPULATIONS

- Upper respiratory disorders
- Tuberculosis
- Skin disorders (athlete's foot) and infestations (scabies, lice)
- Substance use disorders
- HIV/AIDS
- Trauma
- Mental health disorders
- Dental caries
- Hypothermia and heat-related illnesses
- Malnutrition

### STRATEGIES FOR PREVENTING HOMELESSNESS AND ASSISTING INDIVIDUALS WHO ARE HOMELESS

- **Prevent individuals and families from becoming homeless** by assisting them in eliminating factors that can contribute to homelessness.
  - Refer those who have underlying mental health disorders to therapy and counseling.
  - Enhance parenting skills that can prevent young people from feeling the need to run away.
- **Alleviate existing homelessness** by making referrals for financial assistance, food supplements, and health services. Qᵀᶜ
  - Assist homeless clients in locating temporary shelter.
  - Assist clients in finding ways to meet long-term shelter needs.
  - If homeless shelters are not provided in the community, work with government officials to develop shelter programs.

- **Prevent recurrence of poverty, homelessness, and health problems** that result in conditions of poverty and homelessness.
  - Advocate and provide efforts toward political activity to provide needed services for people who have mental health disorders and are homeless.
  - Make referrals for employee assistance and educational programs to allow clients who are homeless to eliminate the factors contributing to their homelessness.

## *Rural residency*

- Rural areas typically have less than 20,000 residents. Frontier areas have less than six persons per square mile.
- Urban areas typically have 20,000 to 49,999 residents, with larger central cities having a population of 1 million people or more.
- In general, low population densities are linked to decreased access to care, decreased health status, and decreased health-seeking behaviors.
- Community health nurses who practice in rural settings often face challenges of limited resources and isolation from other providers. These nurses care for clients who have a broad range of conditions and are at ages across the lifespan.

### HEALTH STATUS OF RURAL RESIDENTS

- Higher infant and maternal morbidity rates
- Higher rates of diabetes mellitus
- Higher rates of obesity
- Less likely to meet physical activity recommendations
- Higher rates of suicide
- Increased trauma/injuries from lightning; farm machinery; drowning and boating; and snowmobile, all-terrain vehicle, and motorcycle crashes
- Increased occupational-associated risks (agriculture, fishing, mining, and construction are the most dangerous industries)
- Less likely to seek preventive care

### BARRIERS TO HEALTH CARE IN RURAL AREAS

- Distance from services
- Lack of personal/public transportation
- Unpredictable weather or travel conditions
- Inability to pay for care (underinsured/uninsured)
- Shortage of rural hospitals/health care providers

### PRIORITY NEEDS FOR RURAL HEALTH

- Cancer prevention and care
- Mental health care
- Substance use prevention and treatment
- Immunization programs
- Family planning

## NURSING INTERVENTIONS FOR RURAL HEALTH

- Assist clients with identifying and applying for assistance programs.
- Use cultural competence when planning interventions.
- Establish trusting partnerships with key individuals in the community.
- Use existing relational ties between residents to foster community outreach initiatives.

# *Migrant employment*

- Seasonal and migrant workers are employed in farming. Employment occurs during the time period required for caring for and harvesting crops.
- Migrant workers make a temporary home during employment at a specific location, and can be paying for their family to live in a different, permanent home at the same time.
- Agricultural workers are not covered under common labor laws (Fair Labor Standards Acts, Occupational Safety and Health Administration protections). Minors 12 years old and older are not covered under the Child Labor Act and can work alongside family members, even under hazardous conditions.
- The Migrant Health Act provides funding for migrant health centers across the U.S., which serve about one-fifth of the migrant worker population.
- Most migrant farmworkers do not speak English as a first language, and can face barriers of discrimination or ineligibility for services. Undocumented workers might not seek services due to fear of deportation.
- The nurse should use cultural competence to design care for individuals and groups of seasonal and migrant workers. Qpcc

## HEALTH PROBLEMS OF MIGRANT WORKERS

- Dental disease
- Tuberculosis
- Chronic conditions
- Stress, anxiety, and other mental health concerns
- Leukemia
- Iron deficiency anemia
- Stomach, uterine, and cervical cancers
- Lack of prenatal care
- Higher infant mortality rates
- STIs, HIV/AIDS

### Pesticide exposure

Pesticide exposure is a significant problem among farm workers. Qs

SUBJECTIVE FINDINGS: Headache, dizziness, dyspnea, nausea, abdominal cramps, poor concentration, eye irritation

OBJECTIVE FINDINGS: Confusion, irritability, muscle weakness and twitching, nasopharyngeal irritation, vomiting, rash

COMPLICATIONS: Long-term exposure is linked to cancer, reproductive problems, Parkinson's disease, liver damage, and behavioral issues. Impaired fetal development can occur among pregnant women exposed to pesticides, even from secondary exposure (contaminated clothing from a family member).

## ISSUES IN MIGRANT HEALTH

- Food insecurity
- Inconsistent income with yearly cycles of unemployment.
- Poor and unsanitary working and housing conditions
- Exposure to environmental pesticides
- Less access to dental, mental health, and pharmacy services
- Inability to afford care
- Reduced availability of services (distance, transportation, hours of service, lack of health record tracking)
- Language barriers and cultural aspects of health care
- Discrimination
- Immigration status (fear that seeking services will lead to deportation)

## STRATEGIES FOR RURAL AND MIGRANT HEALTH CARE

### PRIMARY PREVENTION

- Educate regarding measures to reduce exposure to pesticides (hand washing after working, washing food picked from fields before consumption, changing clothes after work).
- Teach regarding accident prevention measures.
- Provide prenatal care.
- Mobilize preventive services (dental, immunizations).

### SECONDARY PREVENTION

- Create testing programs for tuberculosis and prenatal diagnostic testing.
- Implement screening programs.
  - Pesticide exposure
  - Skin cancer
  - Chronic preventable diseases
  - Communicable diseases
  - Anemia (children)

### TERTIARY PREVENTION

- Treat for manifestations of pesticide exposure.
- Mobilize primary care and emergency services.
- Promote rehabilitation following work-related musculoskeletal injuries.
- Educate clients who have diabetes mellitus or anemia regarding appropriate nutrition.

# Veterans

- The Department of Veterans Affairs (VA) estimates there are 21.6 million veterans in the U.S.
  - Approximately 2 million are women.
  - Approximately 9.9 million are over the age of 65. Ⓖ
- Veterans Health Administration (within the U.S. Department of Veterans Affairs) is responsible for purchasing coverage and delivering health care to veterans and dependents.
  - Nation's largest integrated health care system
  - Inpatient and outpatient services
    - Hospitals
    - Outpatient clinics
    - Home health services
    - Hospice and palliative care services
    - Nursing homes
    - Residential rehabilitation treatment programs
    - Readjustment counseling centers

## VETERAN HEALTH ISSUES

- Mental health (posttraumatic stress disorder, traumatic stress reactions, anger, depression)
- Substance use disorders
- Suicide
- Infectious diseases
- Exposures to herbicides, chemicals, and radiation
- Traumatic brain injuries
- Spinal cord injuries
- Traumatic amputations
- Cold injury
- Military sexual trauma
- Hearing impairments
- Visual impairments

## STRATEGIES FOR VETERAN HEALTH CARE

- Coordinate referrals to available veteran resources.
- Advocate for continued strengthening of the Veterans Health Administration health care system.
- Assist clients to transition from active duty status to veterans.
- Ensure continuity of care between acute and outpatient settings.
- Develop partnerships with local agencies to strengthen resources and achieve mutual goals. Qᴛᴄ

### POSSIBLE STAKEHOLDERS FOR PARTNERSHIPS

- State and local veteran groups
- Offices of rural health
- Local aging services
- Community service organizations
- State and local health departments
- Faith-based organizations
- Public safety departments
- Various media outlets
- Employment services

# Disability

- Disability indicates a factor in the body, senses, or mind that affects the way a person interacts in the daily environment. Exact definitions are determined by specific agencies and groups based on data collection needs.
- Individual or group living environments (unsanitary conditions, poor nutrition, stress), aging, chronic illness, injury, substance use, and genetics can cause physiological or psychological disability.
- Clients who have a disability can use different terminology to describe their condition, including the terms disabled, challenged, or compromised.
- About one-fifth of the U.S. population reports having a disability, some to the extent that it prevents the individual from living alone. Globally, 650 million people have a form of disability.
- The Americans with Disabilities Act was the initial legislation to promote rights for individuals who have a disability.
- The Individuals with Disabilities Education Act (IDEA) also promoted the rights of children who have disabilities and their parents. IDEA ensures free public education and accommodations to prepare the child for independent living, assists with funding of the education, and evaluates the effectiveness of the education. Qᴘᴄᴄ

## EFFECTS OF DISABILITY

- Cost of chronic management
- Decreased employment rates
- Decreased household income and increased poverty rates
- Decreased opportunity for physical activity (physical impairment)
- Isolation and possible self-image issues
- Possible altered roles of family members
- Increased risk for abuse
- Possible inability to live independently
- Presence of comorbidities

## NURSING INTERVENTIONS

The nurse provides care to individuals who have a disability and their families, as well as to groups within the community.
- Implement primary prevention measures to prevent disability (e.g., responsible alcohol use to prevent liver damage).
- Identify disability and chronic disease as early as possible.
- Connect clients with appropriate resources to promote maximum self-care ability.
- Connect families with respite care and counseling.
- Advocate for the rights of individuals, families, and groups dealing with disabilities.
- Ensure public buildings are accessible to individuals who have a physical disability.
- Implement programs to improve quality of life.

# Other at-risk populations

## IMMIGRANTS

- Often have a waiting period to receive financial assistance for medical care
- Unauthorized immigrants are only eligible for immunizations, school lunch, treatment for communicable disease, and emergency care.

### NURSING INTERVENTIONS

- Use cultural competence when planning care.
- Identify risk factors specific to the culture and race.

## REFUGEES

- Forced to leave place of origin due to disaster, war, or threatening environment.
- Eligible for Temporary Assistance for Needy Families, Medicaid, and Supplemental Security Income.

### NURSING INTERVENTIONS

- Assess mental health status and coping following crisis.
- Help individuals apply for assistance programs.

## PREGNANT ADOLESCENTS

- Limited education and job opportunities
- Increased risk for poverty and homelessness
- Increased risk for school problems
- Increased incidence of violence
- Increased risk of malnutrition

### NURSING INTERVENTIONS

- Assist with early identification of pregnant adolescents, including early initiation of prenatal care.
- Provide pregnancy counseling, including alternative courses of action.
- Provide instruction and encouragement in the parenting role in home and peer group-settings.
- Assist in applying for assistance programs (prenatal services, Women, Infants, and Children [WIC]).

## INDIVIDUALS IN THE CORRECTIONAL SYSTEM

- Increased rates of mental health disorders
- Increased incidence of rape and assault in the prison system
- Health care regulated through the Federal Bureau of Prisons (Department of Justice) to promote rights of inmates

### NURSING INTERVENTIONS

- Implement health promotion and counseling during routine care.
- Assist with the design of program to re-integrate individuals into society.
- Foster follow-up with community mental health centers.
- Provide transitional care to reduce the risk of future violent behavior

## LESBIAN, GAY, BISEXUAL, AND TRANSGENDER INDIVIDUALS

- Can face barriers to adequate health care
- State variations in rights for benefits and adoptions
- Can have increased risk for psychological distress and substance use disorders

### NURSING INTERVENTIONS

- Advocate increasing access to care.
- Support the health and functioning of families with LGBT family members. Qpcc
- Provide opportunities for clients to discuss care concerns.

# Application Exercises

1. A nurse at a community clinic is conducting a well-child visit with a preschool-age child. The nurse should identify which of the following manifestations as a possible indication of child neglect? (Select all that apply.)

   A. Underweight

   B. Healing spiral fracture of the arm *ABUSE.*

   C. Genital irritation *ABUSE.*

   D. Burns on the palms of the hands *ABUSE.*

   E. Poor hygiene

2. A nurse is caring for a client who is experiencing alcohol withdrawal. Which of the following findings should the nurse identify as a manifestation of withdrawal?

   A. Decreased blood pressure

   B. Diaphoresis

   C. Pinpoint pupils

   D. Bradycardia

3. A community health nurse is developing an education program on substance use disorders for a group of adolescents. Which of the following information should the nurse include when discussing nicotine and smoking?

   A. Smoking is the fifth-most preventable cause of death in the United States.

   B. Nicotine is a central nervous system depressant.

   C. Withdrawal effects from smoking are minimal.

   D. Tolerance to nicotine develops quickly.

4. A community health nurse is developing strategies to prevent or improve mental health issues in the local area. In which of the following situations is the nurse implementing a tertiary prevention strategy?

   A. Providing support programs for new parents

   B. Screening a client whose partner recently died for suicide risk

   C. Teaching a client who has schizophrenia about medication interactions

   D. Discussing stress reduction techniques with employees at an industrial site

5. A nurse at an urban community health agency is developing an education program for city leaders about homelessness. Which of the following groups should the nurse include as the fastest-growing segment of the homeless population?

   A. Families with children

   B. Adolescent runaways

   C. Intimate partner abuse survivors

   D. Older adults

---

**PRACTICE** Active Learning Scenario

A nurse is reviewing data that will assist with the development of a program to improve health outcomes of vulnerable populations. Use the ATI Active Learning Template: Basic Concept to complete this item.

**RELATED CONTENT:** List at least two national health goals that address vulnerable populations.

**UNDERLYING PRINCIPLES:** List at least three issues that affect vulnerable populations.

**NURSING INTERVENTIONS:** Include at least two strategies to improve access to health care for vulnerable populations.

# Application Exercises Key

1. A. **CORRECT:** Being underweight is a possible manifestation of child neglect.

   B. A healing spiral fracture is a possible manifestation of physical abuse.

   C. Genital irritation is a possible manifestation of sexual abuse.

   D. Burns on the palms of the hands are a possible manifestation of physical abuse.

   E. **CORRECT:** Poor hygiene is possible manifestation of child neglect.

   Ⓝ *NCLEX® Connection: Psychosocial Integrity, Abuse/Neglect*

2. A. Increased blood pressure is a manifestation of alcohol withdrawal.

   B. **CORRECT:** Diaphoresis is a manifestation of alcohol withdrawal.

   C. Dilated pupils are a manifestation of alcohol withdrawal.

   D. Tachycardia is a manifestation of alcohol withdrawal.

   Ⓝ *NCLEX® Connection: Physiological Adaptation, Illness Management*

3. A. Smoking is the leading preventable cause of death in the U.S.

   B. Nicotine is a central nervous system stimulant.

   C. Withdrawal effects from smoking are substantial and increase physical dependence.

   D. **CORRECT:** Tolerance to nicotine does develop quickly.

   Ⓝ *NCLEX® Connection: Health Promotion and Maintenance, High Risk Behaviors*

4. A. The nurse should provide support programs for new parents as a primary prevention strategy.

   B. The nurse should screen a client whose partner recently died for suicide risk as a secondary prevention strategy.

   C. **CORRECT:** Teaching a client who has schizophrenia about medication interactions is a tertiary prevention strategy.

   D. The nurse should discuss stress reduction techniques with employees at an industrial site as a primary prevention strategy.

   Ⓝ *NCLEX® Connection: Health Promotion and Maintenance, Health Promotion/Disease Prevention*

5. A. **CORRECT:** Families with children are the fasting-growing segment of the homeless population.

   B. Adolescent runaways are not the fastest-growing segment of the homeless population.

   C. Intimate partner abuse survivors are not the fastest-growing segment of the homeless population.

   D. Older adults are not the fastest-growing segment of the homeless population.

   Ⓝ *NCLEX® Connection: Health Promotion and Maintenance, Health Promotion/Disease Prevention*

---

## PRACTICE Answer

*Using the ATI Active Learning Template: Basic Concept*

### RELATED CONTENT

- Increase the number of people who have a routine primary care provider.
- Increase the number of people who have health insurance.
- Reduce the number of people who are unable to access or have a delay in accessing health care services and prescribed medications.
- Reduce the number of people who have disabilities who report physical barriers to accessing health and wellness programs in the community.

### UNDERLYING PRINCIPLES

- Violence
- Substance use disorders
- Homelessness
- Mental health issues
- Poverty
- Chronic stress
- Poor self-esteem
- Access to health care services

### NURSING INTERVENTIONS

- Coordinate services at a central location.
- Develop programs that go to the population to deliver health care (home visits, health services bus, on-site clinics).
- Create partnerships to provide free or reduced health care services.
- Advocate for increased availability of health insurance for the uninsured and underinsured.
- Evaluate current health care systems and make recommendations that will strengthen access.
- Collaborate with community leaders to improve/increase the availability of public transportation.
- Ensure the availability of translators with medical training.

Ⓝ *NCLEX® Connection: Health Promotion and Maintenance, Health Promotion/Disease Prevention*

# NCLEX® Connections

When reviewing the following chapter, keep in mind the relevant topics and tasks of the NCLEX outline, in particular:

## Client Needs: Management of Care

**ESTABLISHING PRIORITIES:** Prioritize the delivery of client care.

**LEGAL RIGHTS AND RESPONSIBILITIES:** Report client conditions as required by law.

## Client Needs: Safety and Infection Control

**EMERGENCY RESPONSE PLAN:** Use clinical decision–making/critical thinking for emergency response plan.

**HANDLING HAZARDOUS AND INFECTIOUS MATERIALS:** Follow procedures for handling biohazardous materials.

**STANDARD PRECAUTIONS/TRANSMISSION-BASED PRECAUTIONS/SURGICAL ASEPSIS:** Understand communicable diseases and the modes of organism transmission.

## Client Needs: Physiological Adaptation

**ALTERATIONS IN BODY SYSTEMS:** Provide care to a client with an infectious disease.

**ILLNESS MANAGEMENT:** Apply knowledge of client pathophysiology to illness management.

CHAPTER 6 *Communicable Diseases, Disasters, and Bioterrorism*

Large-scale events have highlighted the need for health care professionals to have knowledge of communicable disease, disaster management, and bioterrorism. Communicable disease is an international health concern.

Nurses have unique skills required to plan for and respond to natural and man-made disasters.

## Communicable diseases

- Worldwide, communicable diseases are responsible for the deaths of millions each year.
- Leading causes of communicable disease deaths include acute respiratory infections (including pneumonia and influenza), HIV/AIDS, diarrheal diseases, tuberculosis, malaria, and measles.
- Other diseases that pose a significant threat to community health include viral hepatitis and sexually transmitted infections. Further information about specific communicable diseases can be found in the *Adult Medical Surgical*, *Maternal Newborn*, and *Nursing Care of Children* Review Modules.
- Community health nurses must maintain knowledge of disease rates, modes of transmission, incubation, early manifestations, periods of communicability, and how to intervene at all levels of prevention related to communicable disease.
- The Centers for Disease Control and Prevention (CDC) recommend routine immunizations according to age. Recommendations include schedules/guidelines for children, adolescents, and adults. A "catch up" schedule and recommendations for health care personnel are also available. The CDC website (www.cdc.gov) provides a high-quality resource for the most current information regarding immunization guidelines. Q EBP

## POPULATIONS AT RISK

- Young children
- Older adults
- Immunosuppressed clients
- Clients who have a high-risk lifestyle
- International travelers
- Health care workers

## MODES OF TRANSMISSION

**Airborne:** inhaled by a susceptible host
- Measles
- Chickenpox
- Tuberculosis (pulmonary or laryngeal)
- Pertussis
- Influenza
- Severe acute respiratory syndrome (SARS)

*[handwritten: MY chicken hez Tb. measles, pertussis, SARS, flu.]*

**Foodborne**
- **Food infection** (bacterial, viral, parasitic infection of food)
  - Norovirus
  - Salmonellosis
  - Hepatitis A
  - Trichinosis
  - *Escherichia coli* (E. coli)
- **Food intoxication** (toxins produced through bacterial growth, chemical contamination, or disease-producing substances)
  - *Staphylococcus aureus*
  - *Clostridium botulinum*

**Waterborne:** fecal contamination of water
- Cholera
- Typhoid fever
- Bacillary dysentery
- *Giardia lamblia*

**Vector-borne:** via a carrier such as a mosquito or tick
- West Nile virus
- Lyme disease
- Rocky Mountain spotted fever
- Malaria

**Direct contact:** transmission of infectious agent from infected host to susceptible host via direct contact
- Sexually transmitted infections: HIV/AIDS, chlamydia, gonorrhea, syphilis, human papilloma virus (HPV), genital herpes, hepatitis B, C, D
- Infectious mononucleosis
- Enterobiasis (pinworms)
- Impetigo
- Lice, scabies

## PORTALS OF ENTRY

- Respiratory passages
- Gastrointestinal tract
- Skin
- Mucous membranes
- Genitourinary tract
- Eyes
- Blood vessels

## PORTALS OF EXIT

- Respiratory secretions
- Feces
- Blood
- Semen
- Vaginal secretions
- Saliva and emesis
- Skin lesion exudates

## DEFENSE MECHANISMS

**Herd immunity:** Protection due to the immunity of most community members making exposure unlikely

**Natural immunity:** Natural defense mechanisms of the body to resist specific antigens or toxins

**Acquired immunity:** Develops through actual exposure to the infectious agent
- **Active:** Production of antibodies by the body in response to infection or immunization with a specific antigen
- **Passive:** Transfer of antibodies to the host either transplacentally from mother to newborn, or through transfusions of immunoglobulins, plasma proteins, or antitoxins

## PREVENTION AND CONTROL Qs

- Prevention and control of communicable disease helps eliminate a disease from a specific location, or completely eradicates the existence of a particular disease.
- Nurses can create community programs that monitor individuals' adherence to treatment regimens to help minimize the spread of disease. This strategy also reduces the risk of complications for individuals, which can reduce the overall burden of disease on a community.
- Public health nurses can use the core functions to target communicable disease. For example, a nurse can identify cases of a disease (assessment), develop a program for city or county government to spray insecticide (policy development), and ensure proper follow-up for individuals who have tuberculin skin testing (assurance).

## COMMUNICABLE DISEASE SURVEILLANCE

- The community health nurse engages in communicable disease surveillance, which includes the systematic collection and analysis of data regarding infectious diseases.
- Descriptive epidemiology is used to investigate disease patterns to identify whom it affected, where the issue is located, how it occurs, why or what the cause is, and when the condition started.
- Information gained from monitoring disease patterns can help identify an unusual disease outbreak or newly emerging disease (public health assessment). The data is also useful in developing public health policies regarding disease management, and to evaluate efficiency of communicable disease programs (assurance).
- Community health nurses can use disease surveillance to track the point of origin of some diseases. For example, the disease can be spread from a common individual or community (host) or a contaminated food or water source (environment).
- Surveillance also helps management of a disease outbreak.
- Reporting of communicable diseases is mandated by state and local regulations, and state notification to the CDC is voluntary.

### NATIONALLY NOTIFIABLE DISEASES
Identified at www.cdc.gov and include the following. Q↳
- Anthrax
- Botulism
- Cholera
- Congenital rubella syndrome (CRS)
- Diphtheria
- Giardiasis
- Gonorrhea
- Hepatitis A, B, C
- HIV infection
- Influenza-associated pediatric mortality
- Legionellosis/Legionnaires' disease
- Lyme disease
- Malaria
- Meningococcal disease
- Mumps
- Pertussis (whooping cough) AIRBORNE
- Poliomyelitis, paralytic
- Poliovirus infection, nonparalytic
- Rabies (human or animal)
- Rubella (German measles)
- Salmonellosis
- Severe acute respiratory syndrome–associated coronavirus disease (SARS-CoV) AIRBORNE
- Shigellosis
- Smallpox
- Syphilis
- Tetanus/C. tetani
- Toxic shock syndrome (TSS) (other than Streptococcal)
- Tuberculosis (TB) AIRBORNE
- Typhoid fever
- Vancomycin-intermediate and vancomycin-resistant *Staphylococcus aureus* (VISA/VRSA)

## HEALTH CARE GOALS

Regarding the control of communicable diseases

### REDUCTIONS IN

- Infections caused by pathogens often transmitted through food
- New HIV diagnoses among adolescents and adults
- New AIDS cases among adolescents and adults
- Number of perinatally acquired HIV and AIDS cases
- Deaths from HIV infection
- Vaccine-preventable diseases (reduction or elimination)
- Number of antibiotic courses for ear infections in young children

### INCREASES IN

- Consumers who follow food safety practices
- Surviving more than 3 years after a diagnosis of AIDS
- Adolescents and adults who have been tested for HIV in the past 12 months
- Testing for HIV in adults who have TB
- Substance use treatment facilities that offer HIV/AIDS education, counseling, and support
- Sexually active persons who use condoms
- Immunization rates among young children
- Immunization rates among adolescents
- Annual seasonal influenza immunizations among children and adults
- Adults who are immunized against pneumococcal disease
- Adults who are immunized against herpes zoster (shingles)
- Tuberculosis clients who complete therapy

## IMMUNIZATION

- The community health nurse plays a major role in increasing immunization coverage to reduce the spread of vaccine-preventable diseases.
- Immunizations are often administered in community health settings, such as public health departments.
- The community health nurse often tracks immunization schedules of at-risk populations, such as children, older adults, immunosuppressed individuals, and health care workers. ⓒ
- The community health nurse must educate the community about the importance of immunizations.
- The community health nurse must stay up to date on current immunization schedule recommendations and appropriate precautions when administering immunizations.

## LEVELS OF PREVENTION

### PRIMARY PREVENTION

- Prevent the occurrence of infectious disease.
- Educate the public regarding the need for immunizations, and federal and state immunization programs.
- Counsel clients traveling to other countries about protection from infectious diseases. Refer clients to the health department for information about mandatory immunizations.
- Educate the public regarding prevention of disease and ways to eliminate risk factors for exposure, such as hand hygiene, universal precautions, proper food handling and storage, use of insecticides, and use of condoms.

### SECONDARY PREVENTION

- Increase early detection through screening and case finding.
- Refer suspected cases of communicable disease for diagnostic confirmation and epidemiologic reporting.
- Provide post-exposure prophylaxis (hepatitis A, rabies).
- Quarantine clients when necessary.
- Use partner notification and contact tracing to identify and screen individuals who have been exposed to a communicable disease. Qs

### TERTIARY PREVENTION

- Decrease complications and disabilities due to infectious diseases through treatment and rehabilitation.
- Monitor treatment compliance, including directly observed therapy (DOT).
- Identify and link clients to needed community resources.

# Disasters

A disaster is an event that causes human suffering and demands more resources than are available in the community. A disaster can be naturally occurring, man-made, or a combination of both, such as a natural disaster causing technological failures.

## LEVELS OF DISASTER MANAGEMENT

### DISASTER PREVENTION (MITIGATION)

- Includes activities to prevent natural and man-made disasters, such as increasing surveillance, improving inspections and airport security, and strengthening public health processes such as immunizations, isolation, and quarantine.
- Activities such as strengthening levees/barriers to prevent flooding and teaching methods of preventing communicable disease transmission are also components.
- The community's threats, vulnerabilities, and capabilities are determined, as are the demographics of community members.
- This level also includes identification and assessment of populations at risk. ⓒ
  - Populations at risk are those that have fewer resources or less of an ability to withstand and survive a disaster without physical harm.
  - These populations tend to be physically isolated, disabled, or unable to access disaster services. Strategic emergency planning is necessary to prevent the loss of lives in susceptible populations.

## DISASTER PREPAREDNESS Qs

- Disaster preparedness occurs at the national, state, and local levels. Personal and family preparedness are crucial components of disaster preparedness, as is professional preparedness for individuals employed in civil service and health care.
- Disaster preparations should stem from threats and vulnerabilities identified in the prevention level, and should coordinate community efforts as well as outline specific roles of local agencies.
- This level of management includes preparedness for natural or man-made disasters.
- Individual and family disaster preparedness include creating an action plan and determining alternative methods of communication, highlighting possible evacuation routes, identifying local and distant meeting places, and creating a disaster kit.
- Setting up a communication protocol is an important part of community disaster planning. The communication plan should provide for access to emergency agencies, such as the American Red Cross, and state and federal government agencies. Qrc
- Disaster drills replicate possible scenarios in the local area and enhance preparedness of community members, government agencies, health care facilities, and businesses.

## DISASTER RESPONSE

- Different agencies, governmental and nongovernmental, are responsible for different levels of disaster response. Some of the agencies with a role in disaster response include the Federal Emergency Management Agency (FEMA), the CDC, U.S. Department of Homeland Security (DHS), American Red Cross (ARC), Office of Emergency Management (OEM), and the public health system.
- Disaster management response includes an initial assessment of the span of the disaster.
  - How many people are affected?
  - How many are injured or dead?
  - How much fresh water and food is available?
  - What are the areas of risk or sanitation problems?
- Disasters are classified according to type, level, and scope.
- If a federal emergency is declared, the National Response Framework (NRF) is activated and provides direction for an organized, effective national response.

## DISASTER RECOVERY

- Recovery begins when danger no longer exists and needed representatives and agencies are available to assist with rebuilding.
- Recovery lasts until the economic and civil life of the community are restored, which can be days, weeks, or even years. At an individual level, it is the time it takes an individual to become functional within a community after a disaster.
- Communicable disease and sanitation controls are important aspects of disaster recovery.
- Post-traumatic stress disorder (PTSD) and delayed stress reactions (DSR) are common during the aftermath of disasters and can affect both caregivers and victims.

## PHASES OF EMOTIONAL REACTION DURING A DISASTER

- **Heroic:** Intense excitement and concern for survival. Often a rush of assistance from outside the area is present.
- **Honeymoon:** Affected individuals begin to bond and relive their experiences.
- **Disillusionment:** Responders can experience depression and exhaustion. Phase contains unexpected delays in receiving aid.
- **Reconstruction:** Involves adjusting to a new reality and continued rebuilding of the area. Counseling is sometimes needed. Those affected begin looking ahead.

# ROLES OF COMMUNITY HEALTH NURSES

## RISK ASSESSMENT

Asking the following questions Qs
- What are the populations at risk within the community?
- Have there been previous disasters, natural or man-made?
- What size of an area or population is likely to be affected in a worst-case scenario?
- What is the community disaster plan?
- What kind of warning system is in place?
- What types of disaster response teams (volunteers, nurses, health care providers, emergency medical technicians, firemen) are in place?
- What kinds of resource facilities (hospitals, shelters, churches, food-storage facilities) are available in the event of a disaster?
- What type of evacuation measures (boat, motor vehicle, train) will be needed?
- What type of environmental dangers (chemical plants, sewage displacement) can be involved?

## DISASTER PLANNING

- Develop a disaster response plan based on the most probable disaster threats.
- Identify the community disaster warning system and communication center, and learning how to access it.
- Identify the community's first responders' disaster plan.
- Make a list of agencies that are available for the varying levels of disaster management at the local, state, and national levels.
- Define the nursing roles in first-, second-, and third-level triage.
- Identify the specific roles of personnel involved in disaster response and the chain of command.
- Locate all equipment and supplies needed for disaster management, including hazmat suits, infectious control items, medical supplies, food, and potable (drinkable) water. Detail a plan to replenish these regularly.
- Check equipment (including evacuation vehicles) regularly to ensure proper operation.
- Evaluate the efficiency, response time, and safety of disaster drills, mass casualty drills, and disaster plans.

## DISASTER RESPONSE

- Activate the disaster management plan.
- Perform triage and direct those affected, coordinating evacuation, quarantine, and opening of shelters.
- Triaging involves identifying those who have serious versus minor injuries, prioritizing care of victims, and transferring those requiring immediate attention to medical facilities.

## DISASTER RECOVERY

- Make home visits and reassess the health care needs of the affected population.
- Provide and coordinate care in shelters.
- Provide stress counseling and assessing for PTSD or delayed stress reactions, and making referrals for psychological treatment.

## EVALUATION OF DISASTER RESPONSE Qɑɪ

- Evaluate the area, effect, and level of the disaster.
- Create ongoing assessment and surveillance reports.
- Evaluate the efficiency of the disaster response teams.
- Estimate the length of time for recovery of community services, such as electricity and running potable water.

# *Bioterrorism*

## AGENTS OF BIOTERRORISM

### CATEGORY A BIOLOGICAL AGENTS

- The highest priority agents, posing a risk to national security because they are easily transmitted and have high mortality rates.
- Examples include smallpox, botulism, anthrax, tularemia, viral hemorrhagic fevers (e.g., Ebola), and plague.

### CATEGORY B BIOLOGICAL AGENTS

- The second-highest priority because they are moderately easy to disseminate, and have high morbidity rates and low mortality rates.
- Examples include typhus fever, ricin toxin, diarrheagenic *E. coli*, and West Nile virus.

### CATEGORY C BIOLOGICAL AGENTS

- The third-highest priority, comprising emerging pathogens that can be engineered for mass dissemination because they are easy to produce, and/or have a potential for high morbidity and mortality rates.
- Examples include hantavirus, influenza virus, tuberculosis, and rabies virus.

## BIOTERRORISM INCIDENTS

### *Inhalational anthrax*

**MANIFESTATIONS**
- Headache
- Fever and chills
- Muscle aches
- Chest discomfort
- Severe dyspnea
- Shock

**PREVENTION**
- Anthrax vaccine for those at high-risk for exposure to anthrax.
- Ciprofloxacin and doxycycline are recommended by the CDC for prevention of anthrax following exposure.

**TREATMENT:** Antitoxin and IV antibiotics are administered if manifestations of an anthrax infection are present.

### *Botulism*

**MANIFESTATIONS**
- Double or blurred vision
- Slurred speech
- Difficulty swallowing
- Progressive muscle weakness
- Difficulty breathing

**PREVENTION:** No approved vaccine

**TREATMENT**
- Airway management with possible mechanical ventilation
- Administration of antitoxin

**ELIMINATION OF TOXIN:** Induction of vomiting, enemas, surgical excision of wound tissue

**SUPPORTIVE CARE:** Nutrition, fluids, prevent complications

### *Smallpox*

**MANIFESTATIONS**
- High fever
- Fatigue
- Head and body aches
- Rash that begins on face and tongue; quickly spreads to the trunk, arms, and legs, then hands and feet; then turns to pus-filled lesions
- Vomiting

**PREVENTION**
- Vaccine for those at high-risk (provides 10 years of immunity); can vaccinate within 3 days of exposure
- Contact and airborne precautions

**TREATMENT:** No cure

**SUPPORTIVE CARE:** Hydration, pain medication, antipyretics, antibiotics for secondary infections

## Ebola

**MANIFESTATIONS**
- Fever
- Severe headache
- Joint and muscle aches
- Fatigue and weakness
- Hemorrhage
- Vomiting and diarrhea
- Shock

**PREVENTION**
- No approved vaccine available
- Don impermeable gown or coverall; disposable gloves (two pairs), boot covers, and apron; and N95 mask. Recommend a second caregiver supervise doffing. Maintain droplet isolation precautions.

**TREATMENT**
- Supportive care IV fluids, dialysis, airway management, psychological counseling.
- Minimize invasive procedures.

## Plague

**MANIFESTATIONS**
These forms can occur separately or in combination.
- **Pneumonic plague:** fever, headache, weakness, pneumonia with shortness of breath, chest pain, cough, and bloody or watery sputum
- **Bubonic plague:** swollen, tender lymph nodes, fever, headache, chills, and weakness
- **Septicemic plague:** fever, chills, weakness, prostration, abdominal pain, shock, disseminated intravascular coagulation (DIC), gangrene of nose and digits

**PREVENTION**
- Vaccine no longer available in the U.S.
- Contact precautions till decontaminated
- Droplet precautions till 72 hr after antibiotics

**TREATMENT:** Gentamicin and fluoroquinolones

## Tularemia

**MANIFESTATIONS**
- Sudden fever, chills, headache, diarrhea, muscle aches, joint pain, dry cough, progressive weakness
- If airborne, life-threatening pneumonia and systemic infection

**PREVENTION:** Vaccine under review by the Food and Drug Administration but not currently available

**TREATMENT**
- Streptomycin or gentamicin is the antibiotic of choice.
- In mass causality, use doxycycline or ciprofloxacin.

## DELIVERY MECHANISMS FOR BIOLOGICAL AGENTS

- Direct contact (subcutaneous anthrax)
- Simple dispersal device (airborne, nuclear)
- Water and food contamination
- Droplet or blood contact

## ROLE OF THE COMMUNITY HEALTH NURSE

- Participate in planning and preparation for immediate response to a bioterrorism event.
- Identify potential biological agents for bioterrorism.
- Survey for and report bioterrorism activity (usually to the local health department).
- Promptly participate in measures to contain and control the spread of infections resulting from bioterrorism activity.

## ASSESSMENT OF THREAT Qs

- Is the population at risk for sudden high disease rates?
- Is the vector that normally carries a specific disease available in the geographical area affected?
- Is there a potential delivery system within the community?

## RECOGNITION OF A BIOTERRORISM EVENT

- Is there a rapidly increasing disease incidence in a normally healthy population?
- Is a disease occurring that is unusual for the area?
- Is an endemic occurring at an unusual time? For example, is there an outbreak of influenza in the summer?
- Are there large numbers of people dying rapidly with similar presenting manifestations?
- Are there any individuals presenting with unusual manifestations?
- Are there unusual numbers of dead or dying animals, unusual liquids/vapors/odors?

## LEVELS OF PREVENTION

**PRIMARY PREVENTION:** Bioterrorism planning
- Prepare with bioterrorism drills, vaccines, and ensuring availability of antibiotics for exposure prophylaxis.
- Design a bioterrorism response plan using the most probable biological agent in the local area.
- Identify the chain of command for reporting bioterrorism attacks.
- Define the nursing roles in the event of a bioterrorism attack.
- Set up protocols for different levels of infection control and containment.

**SECONDARY PREVENTION:** Early recognition
- Activate bioterrorism response plan in response to a bioterrorism event.
- Immediately implement infection control and containment measures, including decontamination, environmental disinfection, protective equipment, community education/notification, and quarantines.
- Screen the population for exposure, assessing rates of infection and administering vaccines as available.
- Assist with and educate the population regarding identification of manifestations and management (immunoglobulin, antiviral, antitoxins, and antibiotic therapy, depending on the agent).
- Monitor mortality and morbidity.

**TERTIARY PREVENTION:** Rehabilitation of survivors
- Monitor medication regimens and referrals.
- Evaluate effectiveness and timeliness of the bioterrorism plan.

# Application Exercises

1. A nurse is preparing a community health program on communicable diseases. When discussing modes of transmission, the nurse should include which of the following illnesses as airborne?

   A. Cholera

   B. Malaria

   C. Influenza

   D. Salmonellosis

2. A home health nurse is discussing portals of entry with a group of newly hired assistive personnel. Which of the following locations should the nurse include as a portal of entry? (Select all that apply.)

   A. Respiratory secretions

   B. Skin

   C. Genitourinary tract

   D. Saliva

   E. Mucous membranes

3. A newly hired public health nurse is familiarizing himself with the levels of disaster management. Which of the following actions is a component of disaster prevention?

   A. Outlining specific roles of community agencies

   B. Identifying community vulnerabilities

   C. Prioritizing care of individuals

   D. Providing stress counseling

4. A community health nurse is educating the public on the agents of bioterrorism. Which of the following agents should the nurse include as Category A biological agents? (Select all that apply.)

   A. Hantavirus

   B. Typhus

   C. Plague

   D. Tularemia

   E. Botulism

5. A community health nurse is determining available and needed supplies in the event of a bioterrorism attack. The nurse should be aware that community members exposed to anthrax will need access to which of the following medications?

   A. Metronidazole

   B. Ciprofloxacin

   C. Zanamivir

   D. Fluconazole

---

### PRACTICE Active Learning Scenario

A community health nurse is responding to a man-made disaster in the local community. Use the ATI Active Learning Template: Basic Concept to complete this item.

**UNDERLYING PRINCIPLES**

- Include three agencies involved in disaster response.
- List two questions to ask to determine the disaster's scope.

**NURSING INTERVENTIONS:** Explain four disaster response nursing roles.

# Application Exercises Key

1. A. Cholera is waterborne illness.

   B. Malaria is a vector-borne illness.

   C. **CORRECT:** Influenza is an airborne illness.

   D. Salmonellosis is a foodborne illness.

   Ⓝ *NCLEX® Connection: Safety and Infection Control, Standard Precautions/Transmission–Based Precautions/Surgical Asepsis*

2. A. Respiratory secretions are a portal of exit.

   B. **CORRECT:** Skin is a portal of entry.

   C. **CORRECT:** The genitourinary tract is a portal of entry.

   D. Saliva is a portal of exit.

   E. **CORRECT:** Mucous membranes are a portal of entry.

   Ⓝ *NCLEX® Connection: Safety and Infection Control, Standard Precautions/Transmission–Based Precautions/Surgical Asepsis*

3. A. Outlining specific roles of community agencies is a component of disaster preparedness.

   B. **CORRECT:** Identifying community vulnerabilities is a component of disaster prevention.

   C. Prioritizing care of individuals is a component of disaster response.

   D. Providing stress counseling is a component of disaster recovery.

   Ⓝ *NCLEX® Connection: Safety and Infection Control, Emergency Response Plan*

4. A. Hantavirus is a Category C biological agent.

   B. Typhus is a Category B biological agent.

   C. **CORRECT:** Plague is a Category A biological agent.

   D. **CORRECT:** Tularemia is a Category A biological agent.

   E. **CORRECT:** Botulism is a Category A biological agent.

   Ⓝ *NCLEX® Connection: Safety and Infection Control, Emergency Response Plan*

5. A. Metronidazole is used to treat trichomoniasis, skin infections, and septicemia.

   B. **CORRECT:** Community members exposed to anthrax will need access to ciprofloxacin. This medication is used for the prophylactic treatment of anthrax.

   C. Zanamivir is used to treat influenza.

   D. Fluconazole is used to treat candidiasis.

   Ⓝ *NCLEX® Connection: Safety and Infection Control, Emergency Response Plan*

---

## PRACTICE Answer

*Using the ATI Active Learning Template: Basic Concept*

### UNDERLYING PRINCIPLES

Involved agencies
- FEMA
- CDC
- U.S. Department of Homeland Security
- American Red Cross
- Office of Emergency Management

Disaster scope
- How many people are affected?
- How many are injured or dead?
- How much potable water and food is available?
- What are the areas of risk or sanitation problems?

### NURSING INTERVENTIONS

- Activate the disaster management plan.
- Perform triage and direct disaster victims.
- Identify people who have serious vs. minor injuries.
- Prioritize care of those affected.
- Transfer those requiring immediate attention to medical facilities.
- Coordinate evacuation or quarantines.
- Open shelters.

Ⓝ *NCLEX® Connection: Safety and Infection Control, Emergency Response Plan*

# ⓝ NCLEX® Connections

When reviewing the following chapter, keep in mind the relevant topics and tasks of the NCLEX outline, in particular:

## Client Needs: Management of Care

**CASE MANAGEMENT:** Provide client with information on discharge procedures to home, or community setting.

**CLIENT RIGHTS:** Advocate for client rights and needs.

**INFORMATION TECHNOLOGY:** Utilize valid resources to enhance the care provided to a client.

**REFERRALS:** Identify community resources for the client.

## Client Needs: Health Promotion and Maintenance

**SELF CARE**
Assess client ability to manage care in the home environment and plan care accordingly.

Consider client self care needs before developing or revising care plan.

# CHAPTER 7

# Continuity of Care

Community health nurses play a large role in maintaining continuity of care for clients as they transition from acute to outpatient settings. Community health nurses use technology to maintain continuity of care.

Community partnerships are essential to improving and maintaining healthy communities. Community health nurses should facilitate the development of partnerships within the community. These partnerships are important in the attainment of collaborative health outcomes.

## EXAMPLES OF PARTNERING ENTITIES

- Individuals
- Families
- Community agencies
- Civic organizations
- Citizen groups
- Educational settings
- Political offices
- Employment bureaus

## CHARACTERISTICS OF SUCCESSFUL PARTNERSHIPS

- Shared power
- Shared goals
- Integrity
- Flexibility
- Negotiation

Groups partnering to elicit needed change in the community are more powerful than a nurse working independently with an individual.

# Referrals, discharge planning, and case management

- A continuum of care assists in coordinating and providing individualized health care services without disruption. The nurse can follow the client from one level of care to the next to ease the client's transition.
- Community health nurses facilitate continuity of care through case management services. These services include focused supervision for individualized care, follow-up, and referrals to appropriate resources. Qpcc
- The establishment of an ongoing relationship between an individual and a health care provider leads to improved health outcomes.

## CONSULTATIONS

A consultant is someone who has specialized knowledge and provides expert advice, services, or information.

### NURSING ACTIONS

- Initiate necessary consults, or notify the provider of the client's needs so the provider can initiate a consult.
- Seek expertise from health care professionals representing a variety of disciplines.
- Request expert opinions of key community members, agency leaders, and other professionals.
- Seek expertise of other nurses, such as specialty nurses (psychiatric nurse, school nurse, gerontological nurse, diabetes management nurse), or advanced practice nurses (psychiatric mental health nurse practitioner, gerontological nurse practitioner).
- Incorporate recommendations from a consultant into the client's plan of care or program planning for the community.
- Coordinate recommendations from multiple consultants (e.g., providers, advanced practice nurses, pharmacists, dietitians, therapists, and holistic providers) to ensure client safety. Qs
- Serve as an expert witness in legal proceedings.
- Serve as a consultant regarding the health care needs of individuals, families, and groups within the community served.

## REFERRALS

- Referrals for individuals in acute care settings typically are based on the medical diagnosis or other relevant clinical information. Resources assist in restoring, maintaining, or promoting health.
- The nurse assists in linking the client with community resources, and must have knowledge of individuals and organizations that can serve as resources. The nurse should also use knowledge of types of assistance the client will accept based on client's personal beliefs and values. Qᴘᴄᴄ
- The nurse educates clients about community resources and self-care measures.

## HEALTH CARE SERVICES

- Providers
- Acute-care settings
- Primary care sites
- Health departments
- Transitional and long-term care facilities
- Home care services
- Rehabilitation services
- Physical therapy services
- Occupational therapy services
- Pharmacies

## SPECIALTY SERVICE AGENCIES

- Support Services
- Psychological services
- Churches
- Support groups
- Life care planners
- Medical equipment providers
- Health insurance companies
- Meal delivery services
- Transportation services

## STEPS IN THE REFERRAL PROCESS

- Engaging in a working relationship with the client
- Establishing criteria for the referral
- Exploring resources
- Accepting the client's decision to use a given resource
- Making the referral
- Facilitating the referral
- Evaluating the outcome

## BARRIERS TO THE REFERRAL PROCESS

### CLIENT BARRIERS
- Lack of motivation
- Inadequate information about community resources
- Inadequate understanding of the need for referral
- Accessibility needs
- Priorities
- Finances
- Cultural factors

### RESOURCE BARRIERS
- Attitudes of health care personnel
- Costs of services
- Physical accessibility of resources
- Time limitations
- Limited expertise working with culturally diverse populations

## FOLLOW-UP CONSIDERATIONS

- Monitor for completion of the referral.
- Assess whether referral outcomes were met.
- Determine if the client was satisfied with the referral.

---

### 7.1 Applying the nursing process during case management

*Assessment*
Clarify the problem by evaluating physical needs, psychosocial issues, functional ability, and financial constraints.

*Diagnosis*
Determine the cause and precipitating factors.

Identify applicable nursing diagnoses based on assessment findings.

*Planning*
In conjunction with the interprofessional team, determine the following.

Prioritization of identified problems

Possible outcomes for the client
- Advantages and disadvantages of possible outcomes
- What role each participant will play in assisting the client to achieve desired outcomes
- Potential effect of the plan on the client

*Implementation*
Contact health care providers.

Provide referral information.

Coordinate all health care services and resources

*Evaluation (continued monitoring)*
Monitor the client to determine whether services are still needed.

Monitor the care provided by the different facilities, comparing against the following.
- Original projected outcomes
- Physical needs
- Psychosocial needs
- Financial needs
- Client and family satisfaction

## DISCHARGE PLANNING

- Discharge planning is an essential component of the continuum of care, and is an ongoing assessment that anticipates the future needs of the client.
- Discharge planning requires ongoing communication between the client, nurse, providers, family, and other members of the interprofessional team. The goal of discharge planning is to enhance the well-being of the client by establishing appropriate options for meeting the health care needs of the client. Qpcc
- Discharge planning begins at admission.

## CASE MANAGEMENT

- Case management nursing is indicated for a variety of health care settings, and includes the following.
  - Promoting interprofessional services and increased client/family involvement
  - Decreasing cost by improving client outcomes
  - Providing education to optimize health participation
  - Reducing gaps and errors in care
  - Applying evidence-based protocols and pathways
  - Advocating for quality services and client rights
- Collaboration between clients, family members, community resources, payer sources, and health care professionals contributes to successful management of the client's health care needs. Qtc
- Case management nurses must possess excellent communication skills in order to facilitate communication among all parties involved. The case management nurse's ability to articulate the needs of the client to various parties can save time and promote successful outcomes.
- Case management nurses can face ethical dilemmas as they liaison between consumers and providers and try to determine the best course of action.
- Legal issues for a case management nurse include making decisions within the legal scope of practice, ensuring referrals are made to providers who are best suited to meet the needs of the client, maintaining confidentiality, and ensuring responsible management of financial charges and spending.
- The nurse uses the nursing process during case management to help the client obtain important services and to treat his condition. (7.1)
- The nurse provides a link between all facets of the health care experience. This means coordinating care among providers, nursing staff, physical and occupational therapists, rehabilitation facilities, home health care, and community resources.
- The case manager must be proactive for the client, balancing the effect of the illness against the cost of care. Increased knowledge of disease processes promotes early intervention and facilitates transition from acute to community-based care.
- Use of community agencies contains costs, because the monitoring of clients leads to better disease management.

## Technology and community nursing

- Technological advances have led to drastic changes in the delivery of health care. The availability of new technologies results in a disruption of old delivery methods, while simultaneously creating new opportunities.
- Some types of technology can assist with cost control. The nurse should consider the expense of new technology compared to potential cost savings prior to implementation for client care.
- The nurse can use technology as a tool to increase awareness and provide education to clients or to collect data (social media campaigns, electronic surveys, use of health literature databases).
- Technology has had an effect on increasing life expectancy, but also can lead to ethical dilemmas in some situations.
- Nurses must remain informed of new technologies in order to deliver optimal care. The introduction of new technologies can have a significant effect on communities, thus influencing health outcomes.

## INFORMATICS AND TELEHEALTH

### Informatics

Informatics is the combination of nursing science with information and communication technologies in the delivery of nursing care. Ql

- Electronic health records (EHR), electronic medical records (EMR), databases, and billing are commonly used within the current health care industry. Hand-held computers and smartphones, geographic information systems, and the Internet all play a role in the delivery of health care.
- Interprofessional teams and clients can hold meetings electronically. Nurses can use chat rooms and asynchronous discussions as alternative delivery methods for client health education, to facilitate support groups, as a mechanism of peer collaboration, or in staff orientations/training.

### Telehealth

Telehealth is the delivery of quality health care through the use of technology.

- Telehealth is particularly useful in rural areas. The ability to deliver specialized, skilled nursing through communication systems that transfer information easily between providers improves access to health care.
- Home care services are increasingly using telehealth technologies in the delivery of client care. Emerging technology allows nurses to provide care to clients at home, while working from a central location such as an office or health care agency. However, with the use of telehealth, it is important to balance the use of these services with actual hands-on care. A combination of these services is needed for optimal client outcomes.

- Agencies transmitting or storing electronic health data must take measures to ensure confidentiality and security of client information.
- Telecommunication technologies can transmit physical, audio, and visual data.

PHYSICAL DATA
- Blood pressure
- Weight
- Blood oxygenation
- Blood glucose
- Heart rate
- Temperature
- ECG results

AUDIO DATA
- Voice conversation
- Heart sounds
- Lung sounds
- Bowel sounds

VISUAL DATA
- Images of wounds
- Images of surgical incisions

## OTHER USES FOR TECHNOLOGY

- Nurses and the interprofessional team can use technology as an outreach tool to educate the public. For example, public service announcements about intimate partner violence have been used to prevent violence and connect community members with appropriate resources.
- Electronic recordkeeping is widely used in public health to create client clinical records, document services provided, maintain financial records, and for creating and managing organizational plans.

# Partnerships with legislative bodies

- Decisions and actions made by legislative bodies can have profound effects on health. Health policy specifically addresses health issues within public policy.
- Laws related to health care regulate licensing, define scope of practice and negligent care, and can outline responsibilities in specific settings, such as in schools or correctional facilities.
- Nurses should know about the process required to develop or amend laws that affect the health of the public.
- To facilitate needed change, it is important for nurses to stay informed of current policy and laws that influence both the health of the community and nursing practice. Nurses also should advocate for policies that protect public health or offer solutions to community problems. Qα
- Nurses can influence individuals who develop policies through professional communication and present evidence-based solutions to address significant health problems.

## NURSES' ROLE IN HEALTH POLICY

CHANGE AGENTS: Advocate for needed change at the local, state, or federal level.

LOBBYISTS: Persuade or influence legislators. Individuals or professional nursing associations can participate in the lobbying process.

COALITIONS: Facilitation of goal achievement through the collaboration of two or more groups.

PUBLIC OFFICE: Serving society and advocating for change by influencing policy development through public service.

# Application Exercises

1. A nurse is creating partnerships to address health needs within the community. The nurse should be aware that which of the following characteristics must exist for partnerships to be successful? (Select all that apply.)

   A. Being a leading partner with decision-making authority

   B. Flexibility among partners when considering new ideas

   C. Adherence of partners to ethical principles

   D. Varying goals for the different partners

   E. Willingness of partners to negotiate roles

2. A nurse is reviewing the various roles of a community health nurse. Which of the following actions is an example of a nurse functioning as a consultant?

   A. Advocating for federal funding of local health screening programs

   B. Updating state officials about health needs of the local community

   C. Facilitating discussion of a client's ongoing needs with an interprofessional team

   D. Performing health screenings for high blood pressure at a local health fair

3. A case management nurse at an acute care facility is conducting an initial visit with a client to identify needs prior to discharge home. After developing a working relationship with the client, the nurse is engaging in the referral process. Which of the following actions should the nurse take first?

   A. Monitor the client's satisfaction with the referral.

   B. Provide the client information to referral agencies.

   C. Review available resources with the client.

   D. Identify referrals that the client needs.

4. A nurse developing a community health program is determining barriers to community resource referrals. Which of the following factors should the nurse include as an example of a resource barrier?

   A. Costs associated with services

   B. Decreased motivation

   C. Inadequate knowledge of resources

   D. Lack of transportation

5. A nurse is working with a client who has systemic lupus erythematosus and recently lost her health insurance. Which of the following actions should the nurse take in the implementation phase of the case management process?

   A. Coordinating services to meet the client's needs

   B. Comparing outcomes with original goals

   C. Determining the client's financial constraints

   D. Clarifying roles of interprofessional team members

---

## PRACTICE Active Learning Scenario

A nurse manager of a home health agency is preparing an in-service about informatics for a group of newly hired nurses. What should the nurse manager include in this presentation? Use the ATI Active Learning Template: Basic Concept to complete this item.

**RELATED CONTENT**
- Define informatics.
- Define telehealth.

**UNDERLYING PRINCIPLES**
- List two types of transmissible physical data.
- List two types of transmissible audio data.
- List two types of transmissible visual data.

**NURSING INTERVENTIONS:** Include three methods of incorporating technology into health care delivery.

# Application Exercises Key

1. A. Shared power must exist for a partnership to be successful.

   B. **CORRECT:** Flexibility must exist for a partnership to be successful.

   C. **CORRECT:** Integrity must exist for a partnership to be successful.

   D. Shared goals must exist for a partnership to be successful.

   E. **CORRECT:** Negotiation must exist for a partnership to be successful.

   Ⓝ *NCLEX® Connection: Management of Care, Concepts of Management*

2. A. The nurse should identify advocacy as a function of a change agent.

   B. **CORRECT:** Updating officials about community health needs is an example of a nurse functioning as a consultant. Community health nurses serve as a consultant regarding the health care needs of individuals, families, and groups within the community served.

   C. The nurse should identify working with an interprofessional team as a function of a case manager.

   D. The nurse should identify performing health screening as a function of a caregiver.

   Ⓝ *NCLEX® Connection: Management of Care, Performance Improvement (Quality Improvement)*

3. A. The nurse should monitor the client's satisfaction with the referral as part of patient-centered care. However, another action must occur first in the referral process.

   B. The nurse should provide the client with information to referral agencies to enable the client to access needed services. However, another action must occur first in the referral process.

   C. The nurse should review available resources with the client to promote self-determination. However, another action must occur first in the referral process.

   D. **CORRECT:** Using the nursing process, the first action the nurse should take at this point in the referral process is to assess client needs. After gathering client data, the nurse should identify referrals that the client needs and prioritize plans. This allows the nurse and client to focus on specific needs while moving forward in the referral process.

   Ⓝ *NCLEX® Connection: Management of Care, Referrals*

4. A. **CORRECT:** Costs associated with services are an example of a resource barrier to community referrals.

   B. Decreased motivation is an example of a client barrier to community referrals.

   C. Inadequate knowledge of resources is an example of a client barrier to community referrals.

   D. Lack of transportation is an example of a client barrier to community referrals.

   Ⓝ *NCLEX® Connection: Management of Care, Continuity of Care*

5. A. **CORRECT:** Coordinating services to meet the client's needs is an action the nurse should take in the implementation phase of the case management process.

   B. Comparing outcomes with original goals is an action the nurse should take in the evaluation phase of the case management process.

   C. Determining the client's financial constraints is an action the nurse should take in the assessment phase of the case management process.

   D. Clarifying roles of interprofessional team members is an action the nurse should take in the planning phase of the case management process.

   Ⓝ *NCLEX® Connection: Management of Care, Case Management*

---

## PRACTICE Answer

*Using the ATI Active Learning Template: Basic Concept*

### RELATED CONTENT

- Informatics: The combination of nursing science with information and communication technologies in the delivery of nursing care
- Telehealth: The delivery of quality health care through the use of technology

### UNDERLYING PRINCIPLES

Physical data
- Blood pressure
- Weight
- Blood oxygenation
- Blood glucose
- Heart rate
- Temperature
- ECG results

Audio data
- Voice conversation
- Heart sounds
- Lung sounds
- Bowel sounds

Visual data
- Wound images
- Surgical incision images

### NURSING INTERVENTIONS

- Electronic records, databases, and billing
- Internet availability of health information and education
- Electronic meetings and chat rooms
- Asynchronous discussions
- Web-based support groups
- Electronic orientation/training
- Health care access in rural areas

Ⓝ *NCLEX® Connection: Management of Care, Information Technology*

# References

Berman, A., Snyder, S., & Frandsen, G. (2016). *Kozier & Erb's fundamentals of nursing: Concepts, process, and practice* (10th ed.). Upper Saddle River, NJ: Prentice-Hall.

Dudek, S. G. (2014). *Nutrition essentials for nursing practice* (7th ed.). Philadelphia: Lippincott Williams & Wilkins.

Eliopoulos, C. (2014). *Gerontological nursing* (8th ed.). Philadelphia: Lippincott Williams & Wilkins.

Halter, M. J. (2014). *Varcarolis' foundations of psychiatric mental health nursing: A clinical approach* (7th ed.). St. Louis, MO: Saunders.

Hockenberry, M. J., & Wilson, D. (2015) *Wong's nursing care of infants and children* (10th ed.). St. Louis, MO: Mosby.

Ignatavicius, D. D., & Workman, M. L. (2016). *Medical-surgical nursing* (8th ed.). St. Louis, MO: Elsevier.

Lowdermilk, D. L., Perry, S. E., Cashion, M. C., & Aldean, K. R. (2016). *Maternity & women's health care* (11th ed.). St. Louis, MO: Elsevier.

Marquis, B. L., & Huston, C. J. (2015). *Leadership roles and management functions in nursing: Theory and application.* (8th ed.). Philadelphia: Lippincott Williams & Wilkins.

Potter, P. A., Perry, A. G., Stockert, P., & Hall, A. (2013). *Fundamentals of nursing* (8th ed.). St. Louis, MO: Mosby.

Stanhope, M., & Lancaster, J. (2014). *Foundations of nursing in the community* (4th ed.). St. Louis, MO: Mosby.

STUDENT NAME _____

CONCEPT_____ REVIEW MODULE CHAPTER_____

| Related Content | Underlying Principles | Nursing Interventions |
|---|---|---|
| (E.G., DELEGATION, LEVELS OF PREVENTION, ADVANCE DIRECTIVES) | | WHO? WHEN? WHY? HOW? |

STUDENT NAME _____

PROCEDURE NAME _____ REVIEW MODULE CHAPTER_____

## Description of Procedure

## Indications

## Interpretation of Findings

## Potential Complications

**CONSIDERATIONS**

### Nursing Interventions (pre, intra, post)

### Client Education

### Nursing Interventions

# Growth and Development

STUDENT NAME _____

DEVELOPMENTAL STAGE _____   REVIEW MODULE CHAPTER_____

## EXPECTED GROWTH AND DEVELOPMENT

| Physical Development | Cognitive Development | Psychosocial Development | Age-Appropriate Activities |
|---|---|---|---|
| | | | |

## Health Promotion

| Immunizations | Health Screening | Nutrition | Injury Prevention |
|---|---|---|---|
| | | | |

# ACTIVE LEARNING TEMPLATE: *Medication*

STUDENT NAME _____

MEDICATION _____ REVIEW MODULE CHAPTER_____

CATEGORY CLASS_____

## PURPOSE OF MEDICATION

### Expected Pharmacological Action

### Therapeutic Use

### Complications

### Medication Administration

### Contraindications/Precautions

### Nursing Interventions

### Interactions

### Client Education

### Evaluation of Medication Effectiveness

# ACTIVE LEARNING TEMPLATE: *Nursing Skill*

STUDENT NAME _____

SKILL NAME_____ REVIEW MODULE CHAPTER_____

## Description of Skill

## Indications

## CONSIDERATIONS

### Nursing Interventions (pre, intra, post)

## Outcomes/Evaluation

## Client Education

## Potential Complications

## Nursing Interventions

STUDENT NAME _____

DISORDER/DISEASE PROCESS _____ REVIEW MODULE CHAPTER_____

| Alterations in Health (Diagnosis) | Pathophysiology Related to Client Problem | Health Promotion and Disease Prevention |
|---|---|---|
| | | |

**ASSESSMENT**

Risk Factors

Expected Findings

Laboratory Tests

Diagnostic Procedures

**SAFETY CONSIDERATIONS**

**PATIENT-CENTERED CARE**

Nursing Care

Medications

Client Education

Therapeutic Procedures

Interprofessional Care

Complications

STUDENT NAME _____

PROCEDURE NAME _____ REVIEW MODULE CHAPTER_____

## Description of Procedure

## Indications

### CONSIDERATIONS

#### Nursing Interventions (pre, intra, post)

## Outcomes/Evaluation

## Client Education

## Potential Complications

## Nursing Interventions